INTERVENTIONAL SPINE PROCEDURES

A CASE-BASED APPROACH

Editors

Jeremy Simon MD
Clinical Instructor, Rothman Institute
1118 West Baltimore Pike
Media, Pennsylvania, USA

Mitchell Freedman DO
Medical Director
Physical Medicine and Rehabilitation
Rothman Institute
Associate Professor, Physical Medicine and Rehabilitation
Thomas Jefferson University Hospital
Philadelphia, Pennsylvania, USA

Michael J Mehnert MD
Clinical Instructor of Rehabilitation Medicine
Thomas Jefferson Medical College
Department of Physical Medicine and Rehabilitation
Philadelphia, Pennsylvania, USA

Alexander R Vaccaro MD PhD
Vice Chairman and Professor
Department of Orthopedics and Neurosurgery
Thomas Jefferson University
Philadelphia, Pennsylvania, USA

JAYPEE

JAYPEE BROTHERS MEDICAL PUBLISHERS (P) LTD

Philadelphia • New Delhi • London • Panama

Jaypee Brothers Medical Publishers (P) Ltd

Headquarters

Jaypee Brothers Medical Publishers (P) Ltd
4838/24, Ansari Road, Daryaganj
New Delhi 110 002, India
Phone: +91-11-43574357
Fax: +91-11-43574314
Email: jaypee@jaypeebrothers.com

Overseas Offices

J.P. Medical Ltd
83, Victoria Street, London
SW1H 0HW (UK)
Phone: +44-2031708910
Fax: +02-03-0086180
Email: info@jpmedpub.com

Jaypee-Highlights.
Medical Publishers Inc
City of Knowledge, Bld. 237
Clayton, Panama City, Panama
Phone: +1 507-301-0496
Fax: +1 507-301-0499
Email: cservice@jphmedical.com

Jaypee Medical Inc.
The Bourse
111 South Independence Mall East
Suite 835, Philadelphia,
PA 19106, USA
Phone: +1 267-519-9789
Email: jpmed.us@gmail.com

Jaypee Brothers
Medical Publishers (P) Ltd
17/1-B Babar Road, Block-B
Shaymali, Mohammadpur
Dhaka-1207, Bangladesh
Mobile: +08801912003485
Email: jaypeedhaka@gmail.com

Jaypee Brothers
Medical Publishers (P) Ltd
Shorakhute, Kathmandu
Nepal
Phone: +00977-9841528578
Email: jaypee.nepal@gmail.com

Website: www.jaypeebrothers.com
Website: www.jaypeedigital.com

Inquiries for bulk sales may be solicited at: jaypee@jaypeebrothers.com

Interventional Spine Procedures—A Case-based Approach

First Edition: **2014**

ISBN 978-93-5152-169-3

Printed at Replika Press Pvt. Ltd.

Dedicated to

My wonderful wife, Karen Simon, who is the smartest person I know and a dedicated wife, mother and OB/Gyn. She is an unending supply of encouragement, support and inspiration. I also dedicate this book to my beautiful children, Zachary and Rosanna Simon, who had to sacrifice some time with Daddy to let him work on this book. Lastly, to my wonderful parents Alan and Jill Simon, who encouraged me to be the best I could be.

Jeremy Simon

This book is a reflection of the hard work and dedication of Jeremy Simon, Michael Mehnert and the Physical Medicine and Rehabilitation team of the Rothman Institute.

Mitchell Freedman

For the many great teachers, I have had along the way....

Michael J Mehnert

Effective spinal care without the support of pain management physicians specializing in diagnoses, medicinal treatment, physical therapy, diagnostic and interventional injections and behavioral therapy would be nonexistent.

Alexander R Vaccaro

Contributors

Arjang Abbasi DO
Interventional Pain Management and Spine Rehabilitation
Long Island Spine Specialists
Larkfield Road, New York, USA

Zachary Broyer MD
Rothman Institute
925 Chestnut Street
Philadelphia, Pennsylvania, USA

Gary P Chimes MD PhD
Physician, Lake Washington Sports and Spine, Chief Medical Advisor
ActivAided Orthotics
Washington DC, USA

Theodore Conliffe MD
Rothman Institute
925 Chestnut Street
Philadelphia, Pennsylvania, USA

Madhuri Dholakia MD
Rothman Institute
925 Chestnut Street
Philadelphia, Pennsylvania, USA

Natacha Falcon DO
Rothman Institute
925 Chestnut Street
Philadelphia, Pennsylvania, USA

Patrick M Foye MD
Professor and Interim Chair
Physical Medicine and Rehabilitation
Director, Coccyx Pain Center
Rutgers New Jersey Medical School
Newark, New Jersey, USA
Co-Director, Musculoskeletal/Spine/Pain Fellowship, Co-Director, Spine Injection Clinic, University Hospital
Newark, New Jersey, USA

Ari Greis DO
Rothman Institute
925 Chestnut Street
Philadelphia, Pennsylvania, USA

Melissa Guanche MD
Program Development
Chief Resident
Department of Rehabilitation Medicine
Thomas Jefferson University Hospital
Philadelphia, Pennsylvania, USA

Gautam Kothari DO
Rothman Institute
3300 Tillman Drive
Bensalem, Pennsylvania, USA

Gautam Malhotra MD
Attending Physician
Department of Veterans Affairs
Physical Medicine and Rehabilitation Service
East Orange, New Jersey, USA
Clinical Associate Professor
Department of Physical Medicine and Rehabilitation
Rutgers New Jersey Medical School
Newark, New Jersey, USA

Lisa Marino DO
Rothman Institute
925 Chestnut Street
Philadelphia, Pennsylvania, USA

Matthew McAuliffe MD
PGY-3 Resident
Department of Rehabilitation Medicine
Thomas Jefferson University Hospital
Philadelphia, Pennsylvania, USA

Michael J Mehnert MD
Clinical Instructor of Rehabilitation Medicine, Thomas Jefferson Medical College, Department of Physical Medicine and Rehabilitation
Philadelphia, Pennsylvania, USA

Michael Molter DO
Rothman Institute
925 Chestnut Street
Philadelphia, Pennsylvania, USA

Shounuck I Patel DO
Department of Physical Medicine and Rehabilitation
Rutgers New Jersey Medical School
Newark, New Jersey, USA

Jesse A Sally MD
Physician, Medical Rehabilitation Incorporated, Director of Sports Medicine and Acute Rehabilitation
Washington Health System
240, Wellness Way
Washington DC, USA

Ferheen Shamim MD
Chief Resident of Program Development
Department of Rehabilitation Medicine
Thomas Jefferson University Hospital
Philadelphia, Pennsylvania, USA

Jeremy Simon MD
Clinical Instructor, Rothman Institute
1118 West Baltimore Pike
Media, Pennsylvania, USA

Anupam Sinha DO
Rothman Institute
925 Chestnut Street
Philadelphia, Pennsylvania, USA

Kelly Williams DO
Resident
Department of Rehabilitation Medicine
Thomas Jefferson University Hospital
Philadelphia, Pennsylvania, USA

Preface

This book is intended as a teaching tool to reinforce the concepts of common problems encountered in the spine clinic. It presents real case scenarios and emphasizes the importance of a thorough history and physical examination, as well as confirmation via appropriate imaging. The judicious and appropriate use of procedures in spine care cannot be stressed enough. Proper patient selection and realistic goals, as well as the use of a multidisciplinary approach are paramount to patient success. This text may be used in the clinic and as a spring-board for discussion as well, as other treatments may often be considered in select patient presentations.

We hope that you find this text educational and thought-provoking.

Jeremy Simon
Mitchell Freedman
Michael J Mehnert
Alexander R Vaccaro

Acknowledgments

I would like to give special thanks to my right hand and medical assistant Esther Coward, my caring and dedicated nurses Stephanie Graham RN BSN and Merrie Fitzgerald RN, and my awesome X-ray Technician Patricia Chase. All of you played an important role in obtaining pictures and treating my patients with dignity and respect.

I would also like to thank my mentor, friend and former fellowship director Michael Furman MD MS who taught me to be a clinician first and interventionalist second. He also taught me how to thoughtfully approach interventional spine procedures.

Many thanks to M/s Jaypee Brothers Medical Publishers (P) Ltd. New Delhi, India, for their invaluable guidance and support in this endeavor.

Jeremy Simon

Contents

Introduction

As clinician-instructors, we often teach during office hours or in the procedure room. Having a case-based, concise text for reference and to drive home the important teaching points and patient presentations for clinical vignettes serves as an efficient tool. This book is intended to introduce common problems and presentations faced in the practice of interventional spine care.

This text is not intended to be a purely a "how-to" book on interventional procedures. A formal fellowship with experienced and competent instructors is recommended for learning safe and proper technique. This text is also not meant to suggest that all patients with these presentations should have a procedure as a treatment. Appropriate non-invasive conservative care and careful patient selection is paramount to ethical care. In addition, procedures performed for pain should be used judiciously and presented as therapeutic options, not as the only method of treatment.

As a clinician and a teacher, having texts for medical students, residents and fellows to refer is very helpful to direct their learning. There are several excellent and comprehensive books for reinforcing interventional techniques in spine care. There are excellent texts that give detailed background information and in-depth discussions regarding pathophysiology and pharmacology.

The purpose of this text is to allow the clinician-instructor to present a typical pain pattern, patient history and physical examination findings with appropriate imaging and their interpretation. We emphasize the importance of the history and physical examination, as well as alternative treatment options.

All of the contributors in this book practice musculoskeletal medicine and these vignettes represent real patients in our practices. The bolded type in the physical examination section is intended to emphasize clues to making the diagnosis.

We hope that you find this text to be educational and informative.

Basic Principles of Fluoroscopically-guided Procedures

1

Jeremy Simon

INTRODUCTION

Interventional procedures in the treatment of pain have become a common practice. While the use of fluoroscopy can significantly reduce the risk of complications, some basic principles must be utilized to reduce the potential for harm. The practitioner should be well-educated and competent in anatomy, fluoroscopic anatomy and in needle-driving to safely deliver the treatment. It is recommended that a formal fellowship with an experienced clinician(s) be performed before using these procedures in clinical practice.

Ultimately these are elective procedures. The principle of *Primum non nocere*, "first do no harm" must be considered in patient selection. This applies to the patient's ability to stop anticoagulants, poor experiences with prior injections, glycemic control, and degree of neurologic impairment. The author will not perform cervical interlaminar epidural injections in patients with signs and symptoms of myelopathy, cord edema, or significant cord compression as demonstrated by the lack of cerebrospinal fluid around the cervical spinal cord on axial X-rays. This is for fear of placing pressure on a tenuous spinal cord and potential reversible or irreversible cord damage.[1] While other practitioners may differ in their opinion on this matter, the concept of "do no harm" should always be considered when planning any interventional procedure.

STERILE PREPARATION

Thorough handwashing or scrubbing should be performed prior to gloving. Sterile gloves should be utilized and put on the hands without touching the outer portion with the ungloved fingers.

A sterile field consists of a preparation of the skin with a povidone solution or chlorhexidine. Some studies showed superiority of chlorhexidine[2-6] while others have shown no difference.[7-11] The preparation should be made after locating the area with a spot film and making concentric circles from the target area outward. This reduces the chance of "inoculating" the target region with bacteria present on other areas of the skin. The area should be allowed to dry prior to skin puncture. A fenestrated sterile drape or sterile towels should be placed around the target area.

The use of sterile medications from an FDA-regulated (Food and Drug Administration regulated) pharmaceutical company is a must. Reports of fungal meningitis from presumed sterile medications have made it imperative to obtain medications from well-vetted companies.[12-14] Medications should be drawn in a sterile fashion at the time of the procedure and placed in the sterile tray.

NEEDLE-DRIVING

The spinal needle has a notch at the top and a beveled tip. The inner portion, or cannula, is removable and gives added stiffness to the needle as well as helps to prevent tissue from entering the needle during placement. The tendency of the needle is to move in the direction of the slope of the bevel. Tissue will deflect against the bevel. This is the "opposite" direction as the notch. For example, if the notch is up, the tendency of the needle is to go down. If it is facing left, it will "tend" to go right.

The further the needle is into tissue, particularly stiffer tissues such as muscle, it will be more difficult to direct. Many practitioners will "accentuate the bevel" by placing a bend on the needle of about 10 degrees. This allows for larger movements to be made in deeper tissues.

Tuohy needles utilized in interlaminar approaches are of typically larger bore, often 18- or 20-gauge. They are thus more difficult to steer in tissue. The bevel and notch are in the same orientation, i.e. the needle will tend to move in the "same" direction as the notch.

FLUOROSCOPY

The use of fluoroscopy adds a significant advantage in procedural safety. The use of an anterior-posterior (AP) and lateral views allow the practitioner to determine the precise location of the needle before administering the treatment. The AP view lets the practitioner how close to the midline, or how "medial" the needle tip is placed. The lateral view shows the depth of the needle. This allows for subtle adjustments so that the needle can be placed accurately and without violation of the spinal canal.

Care should be exercised by the interventionalist to minimize their exposure to radiation in the procedure suite. Radiation badges and rings should be worn and monitored to keep record of year-to-date and lifetime exposure. Lead aprons should be used to keep the soft-tissues, particularly the gonads and thyroid, covered. X-ray reducing goggles should also be worn to minimize eye exposure. X-ray reducing gloves may also be worn underneath the sterile gloves when possible.

Planning the procedure ahead of time by noting on plain films and magnetic resonance imaging (MRI)/computed tomography (CT) scan if there is transition anatomy (lumbarization of S1, sacralization of L5), hardware, osteophytes or obesity may also allow for reduced fluoroscopy times. A study in obese individuals showed a significantly longer fluoroscopy times in obese individuals.[15]

The use of pulsed, intermittent and half-dose fluoroscopy can reduce exposures, particularly at noncritical portions of the placement of the needle. Reducing the fluoroscopy time is also useful in so far as patient and procedure safety are not compromised.

The top of the C-arm is known as the image intensifier and the bottom is the source of the X-ray. Keeping farther away from the source when possible will reduce the interventionalist's exposure, as well as the "scatter" of the X-ray from the patient. The X-ray exposure will decrease as an "inverse square" of the distance from the source.[16] Placing lead over the patient in areas outside of the field, when practical, may reduce scatter.[17]

Potential risks of radiation exposure include cataracts, radiation burns and various types of cancers.[18] These risks are cumulative and monthly readings are essential for helping to alert the practitioner of their exposure.

Parallax

Maximizing safety, minimizing risk and improving accuracy are all part of advantages in the use of fluoroscopy in interventional spine procedures. Knowing how to position the patient and how to obtain ideal images in set-up helps also to expedite the procedure and reduce patient discomfort through reducing needle manipulation.

The top of the fluoroscopy unit, the image intensifier, can be thought of as the physician's eyes. The picture on the screen represents the X-ray image of the segment at that angle. If the needle is placed in line with the beam, it will appear as a dot with the hub of the needle visible (Fig. 1.1). "Following the beam", or following this target trajectory, allows for minimal needle manipulation. The concept of aligning the needle with the X-ray beams is also known as "parallax".

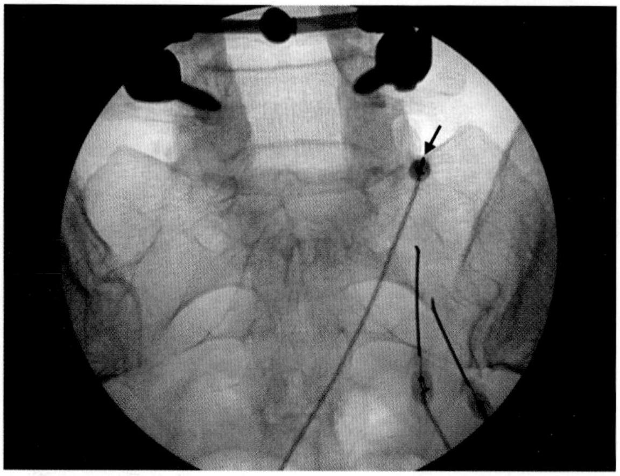

Fig. 1.1: Sacroiliac denervation. Note the needle over the right L5 dorsal ramus is seen in parallax, while the needles placed below are not

CONTRAST

Nonionic iodinated contrast allows the interventionalist to confirm that the medication is placed in the desired location. The use of extension tubing allows for the live injection of contrast while keeping the hands out of the field and reducing X-ray exposure. While aspiration of blood is a specific indicator of vascular placement, it is not sensitive.[19,20]

Patients with known allergy to iodine need to have proper medication prophylaxis and monitored during and after the procedure (see Chapter 15: Adverse Reactions to Medications). Attempts to minimize the amount of contrast injected should be made within reason.

ANTICOAGULANTS

Differing opinions exist regarding the cessation of anticoagulants during interventional spine procedures. Spinal injections in fully anticoagulated-patients are generally contraindicated.[21,22] Clearance from the prescribing physician is essential, and the risks and benefits need to be weighed by both physicians prior to scheduling the procedure.

Nonsteroidal anti-inflammatory agents are generally accepted to be safe for most nonsurgical interventional spine procedures.[23] A survey of interventional pain physicians showed that most held antithrombotics prior to procedures and fewer held nonsteroidal anti-inflammatory drugs (NSAIDs).[24] While not a standard, below is the author's practice's anticoagulation protocol.

Protocol for Holding Anticoagulants[25-27]

The following anticoagulant holding schedule is recommended prior to spinal procedures (clearance must be obtained from the prescribing physician first):

- *Ticlopidine (Ticlid)*: Hold for 14 days
- *Aspirin*: Hold for 7 days
  - including: Alka-Seltzer, Anacin, Fiorinal, Ascriptin, Bayer, Bufferin, Lortab ASA, Darvon, Ecotrin, Excedrin, Percodan, Midol, Pepto-Bismol, Talwin
- *Clopidogrel (Plavix)*: Hold for 7 days
- *Dipyridamole (Aggrenox or Persantine)*: Hold for 7 days
- *Cilostazol (Pletal)*: Hold for 7 days
- *Pentoxifylline (Trental)*: Hold for 7 days
- *Agrylin (Anagrelide)*: Hold for 7 days
- *Prasugrel (Effient)*: Hold for 7 days
- *Ticagrelor (Brilinta)*: Hold for 7 days
- *Warfarin (Coumadin)*: Hold for 5 days
  - INR (drawn day before or day of procedure) should be below 1.3 to proceed with injection
- *Dabigratan (Pradaxa)*: Hold for 5 days
- *Rivaroxaban (Xarelto)*: Hold for 5 days
- *Apixaban (Eliquis)*: Hold for 5 days
- *NSAIDs*: Hold for 5 days for cervical and thoracic procedures. Does not need to be held for lumbar and hip procedures
  - including: Diclofenac, Etodolac, Fenoprofen, Flurbiprofen, Ibuprofen, Indomethacin, Ketoprofen, Ketorolac, Meloxicam, Nabumetone, Naproxen, Oxaprozin, Piroxicam, Sulindac, Celebrex
- *Fondaparinux (Arixtra)*: Hold for 24–48 hours
- *Enoxaparin (Lovenox)*: Hold for 12 hours (prophylactic dose) or 24 hours (therapeutic dose)
- *Heparin*: Hold for 4 hours.

Herbal drugs (specifically garlic, ginseng and gingko) seem to represent no added significant risk for the development of spinal hematoma in patients having epidural or spinal anesthesia.

REFERENCES

1. Hodges SD, Castleberg RL, Miller T, et al. Cervical epidural steroid injection with intrinsic spinal cord damage. Two case reports. Spine. 1998;23:2137-42; discussion 2141-2.
2. Clevenot D, Robert S, Debaene B, et al. Critical review of the literature concerning the comparative use of two antiseptic solutions before intravascular or epidural catheterization. Annales francaises d'anesthesie et de reanimation. 2003; 22:787-97.

3. Yeung LL, Grewal S, Bullock A, et al. A comparison of chlorhexidine-alcohol versus povidone-iodine for eliminating skin flora before genitourinary prosthetic surgery: a randomized controlled trial. The Journal of Urology. 2013;189:136-40.
4. Dumville JC, McFarlane E, Edwards P, et al. Preoperative skin antiseptics for preventing surgical wound infections after clean surgery. Cochrane Database of Systematic Reviews. 2013; 3:CD003949.
5. Krobbuaban B, Diregpoke S, Prasan S, et al. Alcohol-based chlorhexidine vs. povidone iodine in reducing skin colonization prior to regional anesthesia procedures. Journal of the Medical Association of Thailand—Chotmaihet Thangphaet. 2011;94:807-12.
6. Kinirons B, Mimoz O, Lafendi L, et al. Chlorhexidine versus povidone iodine in preventing colonization of continuous epidural catheters in children: a randomized, controlled trial. Anesthesiology. 2001; 94:239-44.
7. Rugpolmuang L, Thanabodeethada R, Riansuwan K. Comparison of the effectiveness in bacterial decontamination between chlorhexidine gluconate and povidone-iodine solution in foot and ankle: a pilot study. Journal of the Medical Association of Thailand—Chotmaihet Thangphaet. 2012;95(Suppl 9): S95-8.
8. Girard R, Comby C, Jacques D. Alcoholic povidone-iodine or chlorhexidine-based antiseptic for the prevention of central venous catheter-related infections: in-use comparison. Journal of Infection and Public Health. 2012;5:35-42.
9. Caldeira D, David C, Sampaio C. Skin antiseptics in venous puncture-site disinfection for prevention of blood culture contamination: systematic review with meta-analysis. The Journal of Hospital Infection. 2011;77:223-32.
10. Sistla SC, Prabhu G, Sistla S, et al. Minimizing wound contamination in a 'clean' surgery: comparison of chlorhexidine-ethanol and povidone-iodine. Chemotherapy. 2010;56:261-7.
11. Kasuda H, Fukuda H, Togashi H, et al. Skin disinfection before epidural catheterization: comparative study of povidone-iodine versus chlorhexidine ethanol. Dermatology. 2002;204 (Suppl 1): 42-6.
12. Bell BP, Khabbaz RF. Responding to the outbreak of invasive fungal infections: the value of public health to Americans. JAMA. 2013;309:883-4.
13. Smith RM, Schaefer MK, Kainer MA, et al. Fungal infections associated with contaminated methylprednisolone injections–Preliminary Report. The New England Journal of Medicine; 2012.
14. Kainer MA, Reagan DR, Nguyen DB, et al. Fungal infections associated with contaminated methylprednisolone in Tennessee. The New England Journal of Medicine. 2012;367:2194-203.
15. Smuck M, Zheng P, Chong T, et al. Duration of fluoroscopic-guided spine interventions and radiation exposure is increased in overweight patients. PM & R: The Journal of Injury, Function, and Rehabilitation. 2013;5:291-6.
16. Shafiei SA, Hassanzadeh H. A simple calculation method for determination of equivalent square field. Journal of Medical Physics/Association of Medical Physicists of India. 2012;37:107-11.
17. Manchikanti L, Cash KA, Moss TL, et al. Effectiveness of protective measures in reducing risk of radiation exposure in interventional pain management: a prospective evaluation. Pain Physician. 2003;6:301-5.

18. Brenner DJ, Doll R, Goodhead DT, et al. Cancer risks attributable to low doses of ionizing radiation: assessing what we really know. Proceedings of the National Academy of Sciences of the United States of America. 2003;100:13761-6.
19. Furman MB, O'Brien EM, Zgleszewski TM. Incidence of intravascular penetration in transforaminal lumbosacral epidural steroid injections. Spine. 2000; 25:2628-32.
20. Furman MB, Giovanniello MT, O'Brien EM. Incidence of intravascular penetration in transforaminal cervical epidural steroid injections. Spine. 2003;28:21-5.
21. Gogarten W, Vandermeulen E, Van Aken H, et al. Regional anaesthesia and antithrombotic agents: recommendations of the European Society of Anaesthesiology. European Journal of Anaesthesiology. 2010;27:999-1015.
22. Millar FA, Mackenzie A, Hutchison G, et al. Hemostasis-altering drugs and central neural block. A survey of anesthetic practice in Scotland and the United Kingdom. Regional Anesthesia. 1996;21:529-33.
23. Horlocker TT, Bajwa ZH, Ashraf Z, et al. Risk assessment of hemorrhagic complications associated with nonsteroidal antiinflammatory medications in ambulatory pain clinic patients undergoing epidural steroid injection. Anesthesia and Analgesia. 2002;95:1691-7, table of contents.
24. Manchikanti L, Benyamin RM, Swicegood JR, et al. Assessment of practice patterns of perioperative management of antiplatelet and anticoagulant therapy in interventional pain management. Pain Physician. 2012;15:E955-68.
25. Horlocker TT, Wedel DJ, Rowlingson JC, et al. Regional anesthesia in the patient receiving antithrombotic or thrombolytic therapy: American Society of Regional Anesthesia and Pain Medicine Evidence-Based Guidelines (Third Edition). Regional Anesthesia and Pain Medicine. 2010;35:64-101.
26. Horlocker TT, Wedel DJ, Rowlingson JC, et al. American College of Chest P. Executive summary: regional anesthesia in the patient receiving antithrombotic or thrombolytic therapy: American Society of Regional Anesthesia and Pain Medicine Evidence-Based Guidelines (Third Edition). Regional Anesthesia and Pain Medicine. 2010;35:102-5.
27. Ortel TL. Perioperative management of patients on chronic antithrombotic therapy. Hematology/American Society of Hematology Education Program. 2012;2012:529-35.

Lumbar Disc Herniation with Radiculopathy: Selective Spinal Nerve Injection

2

Lisa Marino, Jeremy Simon

CHIEF COMPLAINT

The patient complains about lower back pain and left thigh pain.

HISTORY OF PRESENTING ILLNESS

A 47-year-old right-handed male presents for consultation with complaints of left-sided low back and buttock pain that radiates into the posterolateral thigh with associated numbness into all five toes of the left foot on plantar and dorsal aspects. He describes his pain as a constant burning type rated at a 9/10 on the numeric pain scale. The pain began 4 months ago after playing 18 holes of golf and became progressively worse. The symptoms are aggravated with standing, walking and lying down. He gets some relief with sitting and medications. He denies fevers, chills, and/or night sweats. There are no associated bowel or bladder symptoms, progressive weakness, saddle anesthesia or night-time pain.

Treatment has consisted of physical therapy for 6 weeks, two fluoroscopically-guided transforaminal epidural injections, hydrocodone and celecoxib. The physical therapy offered no relief of pain. *He underwent two L5 transforaminal epidural injections and received 2–10 days of subsequent pain relief, after which the symptoms returned to baseline.* The pain was interfering with the patient's sleep and ability to work as an elevator repairman. He had a lumbar microdiscectomy at L5-S1 10 years prior with complete resolution of his left lower extremity radicular symptoms until the aforementioned episode. He was referred to a spinal interventionalist by the spine surgeon for a series of diagnostic selective nerve root injections to determine if surgery would be indicated.

PAST MEDICAL/SURGICAL HISTORY

Lumbar microdiscectomy L5-S1 10 years prior

REVIEW OF SYSTEMS

Otherwise negative

FAMILY HISTORY

Mother alive and healthy, father deceased from head and neck cancer.

SOCIAL HISTORY

No alcohol, tobacco or illicit drug history. He is married, with two children. Employed fulltime in elevator repair and construction, no workmen's compensation claims.

CURRENT MEDICATIONS

Celecoxib 200 mg daily, Hydrocodone/apap 10/325 one to two tablets daily to bid prn pain.

ALLERGIES

None

PHYSICAL EXAMINATION

Height: 6′7″, Weight: 275 lbs, Pulse: 84/min, Blood Pressure (BP): 132/88 mm Hg. The patient was pleasant, conversant, well developed, oriented and in no acute distress. Affect and mood were normal. Rapid alternating movement was unremarkable. The patient demonstrated no overt pain behavior and was fully cooperative with the examination. Inspection and palpation did not identify significant misalignment, atrophy or asymmetry in the head, neck, thoracolumbar spine and lower limbs. There was no evidence of dislocation or fracture in the neck, back, and either lower limb. The pelvis was level without evidence of significant scoliosis. The patient had an *antalgic gait favoring left lower extremity weight bearing*. Toe and heel walk were intact. *Lumbar flexion, extension, rotation and side bending range of motion were diminished in all planes by 50% secondary to pain*. Bilateral hip and knee range of motion was grossly functional and symmetric. Strength testing was 5/5 in the hip flexors, extensors, knee flexors, extensors, dorsiflexors, everters, inverters and extensor hallucis longus (EHL) as well as grossly in the neck, spine and pelvis. Sensation to light touch and distal pulses were within normal limits in the lower limbs. The trunk and lower limbs were without evidence of lymphadenopathy, edema or rash. Muscle stretch reflexes were 2+ and symmetric in the knees and ankles without upper motor neuron signs. *Straight leg raise test was negative, but reproduced left thigh pain.*

IMAGING STUDIES

Radiographs of the lumbar spine were reviewed. There were posterior-anterior, lateral, flexion and extension views. Five normal appearing lumbar vertebrae were present without evidence of fracture, spondylolysis or spondylolisthesis. *There was evidence of decreased disc height at the L3-4, L4-5 and L5-S1 levels and evidence of a left hemilaminotomy.*

Magnetic resonance imaging (MRI) of the lumbar spine showed moderate degenerative changes at the L3-4 and L4-5. L5-S1 disc was significantly degenerated. A disc bulge was present at all three lower lumbar levels with lateral recess stenosis at L3-4 and L4-5. L5-S1 had severe bilateral foraminal stenosis with evidence of a hemilaminotomy.

ELECTRODIAGNOSTIC STUDIES

Electromyography (EMG)/Nerve conduction studies (NCS) of the bilateral lower extremities were normal.

DIAGNOSIS

Lumbar radiculopathy

TREATMENT

The patient presented to the clinic with several conservative treatments producing unsuccessful outcomes including medication management, physical therapy and therapeutic spinal interventions. Certainly, in the absence of neurological dysfunction, conservative measures should be tried before surgical intervention. Nonetheless, the patient was significantly limited by pain and was interested in pursuing definitive treatment. Subsequent to surgical consultation, it was determined that if further testing confirmed an L5 radiculopathy surgery would be indicated.

The patient presented with severe left-sided buttock and thigh pain associated with foot numbness. There were several diagnoses that could be the cause of his symptoms including lumbar radiculopathy, sacroiliac joint dysfunction, hamstring tendonitis, lumbar internal disc disruption syndrome with somatic referral and piriformis syndrome, among others. Although symptoms associated with standing and walking are expected with radiculopathy from spinal stenosis, the patient's pain radiated only into a portion of the L5 dermatome, not the classic area below the knee, making the diagnosis of L5 radiculopathy indeterminate.

The physical examination offered little evidence of lumbar radiculopathy. The patient had no dural root tension signs, myotomal weakness or dermatomal patterns of sensory disturbance that is often seen with lumbar radiculopathy.

The normal NCS/EMG was not supportive for ruling in the presence of acute radiculopathy. Electrodiagnostic evidence of radiculopathy can often be absent, with test sensitivity ranging from 49% to 92%.[1] Therefore, the patient's normal study did not exclude a lumbar radiculopathy as a source of his pain. Even if the NCS/EMG showed evidence of a chronic lumbar radiculopathy, it would not be useful given his previous history of lumbar surgery for left-sided lumbar radiculopathy.

The imaging studies showed three lower lumbar discs with abnormalities and varying degrees of lateral recess and foraminal stenosis; any of which could contribute to the patient's symptoms.

The short-term pain relief from the L5 transforaminal injection did not definitively indicate that the L5 nerve root was the pain generator. The L5 transforaminal injection was performed with both steroid and lidocaine and subsequent pain relief could have been a systemic steroid response.

Lumbar internal disc disruption syndrome was a consideration as a source of the patient's pain; therefore lumbar discography could have been an alternate diagnostic procedure. However, the use of discography for accurately pinpointing a pain generator is a controversial topic. In a study by Berg et al. discography was shown to influence surgical decision making in up to 72% of cases, thus supporting its use.[2] Opposing arguments report a best-case positive predicted value for provocative discography to be 50–60%, meaning that a positive discogram does not necessarily correlate with effective pain relief after fusion of the proposed painful disc.[3] Additionally, modern discography methods have been shown to accelerate the degenerative changes of the disc on imaging studies.[4]

In this case, lumbar radiculopathy was the leading differential diagnosis for the patient, however further diagnostic information was desired by the surgeon. Lumbar disc herniation with radiculopathy. Selective nerve root injections in conjunction with a pain diary would help to clarify the presence of an L5 radiculopathy since the other studies and physical examination was equivocal.

Diagnostic selective nerve injections have been used since the 1970s to determine sources of pain and have been shown to provide a sensitivity of 90–95%.[5,6] False positives can occur but can be minimized with appropriate injection technique.[6,7] A diagnostic selective nerve root injection was recommended in this case because less invasive testing was unable to accurately pinpoint the pain generator of the abnormal radicular pattern. The surgeon requested an L3, L4 and L5 diagnostic selective nerve root injection for confirmation of the suspected diagnosis of L5 radiculopathy. A positive diagnostic injection would change treatment, since the patient would be a surgical candidate if pain was relieved with the test injection.

Given the patient's pain distribution into the posterior thigh, an S1 selective nerve block could also be considered. In this case, the selective nerve root injections were requested to determine if surgical intervention would be of benefit. The L3, L4 and L5 nerve roots had the most compressive pathology on MRI making them a potential for decompressive surgical intervention and therefore were the only nerves selected for targeted diagnostic injections.

Diagnostic injections should be performed one nerve level per visit. The patient should complete a pre- and post-injection standard pain drawing and a numeric pain rating scale. The injection should be performed with fluoroscopic guidance and contrast dye confirmation of nerve outline. The spinal nerve and the dorsal root ganglion are the desired target.

In this case, informed consent was obtained and risks of the procedure were reviewed with the patient which include, but were not limited to infection, allergic reaction, nerve damage, paralysis, epidural hematoma, syncope, headache, respiratory or cardiac arrest, worsening pain and scar formation.

Vital signs were monitored prior to, during, and after the procedure.

The patient was placed in the prone position on the fluoroscopy table. The C-arm was rotated to a slightly oblique and ipsilateral position. The lumbar area was prepped and draped in the usual sterile fashion. Next, the L5 neuroforamen was identified under fluoroscopic guidance. A small skin wheel was raised over the insertion site with local anesthetic. Using a sterile technique, a 22-gauge, 3.5-inch spinal needle was inserted into the skin. Under intermittent fluoroscopic guidance, the needle was advanced towards the foramen in the oblique position aiming for the uppermost aspect of the superior articular process and just inferior to the pedicle. Once the needle entered the muscle adjacent to the spine, the C-arm was rotated to the anterior-posterior view. The needle was then advanced into "the safe triangle",[8] inferior to the 6 o'clock position of the pedicle and superolateral to the exiting spinal nerve. The borders of "the safe triangle" are the horizontal base of the pedicle, the traversing nerve as the hypotenuse, and the posterolateral border of the vertebral body. The needle position was checked in the anterior-posterior and lateral positions.

Extension tubing was then attached to the spinal needle and under live fluoroscopy 1–2 milliliters of contrast dye was injected to verify spinal nerve and dorsal root ganglion outline. The injection of contrast medium should be slow, about 1 mL per 20 seconds; this was done to determine the volume

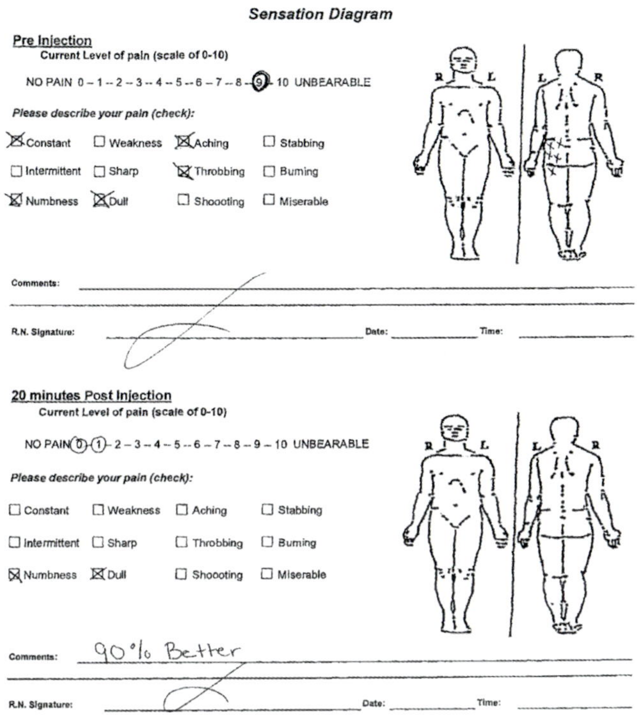
Sensation Diagram

Pre Injection
Current Level of pain (scale of 0-10)
NO PAIN 0 – 1 – 2 – 3 – 4 – 5 – 6 – 7 – 8 – (9) – 10 UNBEARABLE
Please describe your pain (check):
☒ Constant ☐ Weakness ☒ Aching ☐ Stabbing
☐ Intermittent ☐ Sharp ☒ Throbbing ☐ Burning
☒ Numbness ☒ Dull ☐ Shooting ☐ Miserable
Comments:
R.N. Signature: Date: Time:

20 minutes Post Injection
Current Level of pain (scale of 0-10)
NO PAIN (0) – (1) – 2 – 3 – 4 – 5 – 6 – 7 – 8 – 9 – 10 UNBEARABLE
Please describe your pain (check):
☐ Constant ☐ Weakness ☐ Aching ☐ Stabbing
☐ Intermittent ☐ Sharp ☐ Throbbing ☐ Burning
☒ Numbness ☒ Dull ☐ Shooting ☐ Miserable
Comments: 90% Better
R.N. Signature: Date: Time:

Fig. 2.1: Pain diagram pre-selective spinal nerve and post-selective spinal nerve injection performed for the left L5 spinal nerve. Note the patient reports 90% relief of his typical pain

needed to outline the targeted nerve. The volume needed of contrast dye to outline the nerve should be the same volume used for the local anesthetic. The contrast should flow along the surface of the nerve outlining the dorsal root ganglion and the nerve root sleeve. Medially the dye should curve up around the pedicle and laterally should outline the nerve. No vascular uptake, subarachnoid flow, or epidural spread to adjacent levels should be noted on live fluoroscopic views.

After aspiration was negative for return of blood or cerebrospinal fluid, 0.5 mL of 0.25% Bupivacaine was injected. The needle was then removed intact. The area was cleansed and a band-aid was applied to the injection site.

Twenty minutes after the injection, the patient completed the post-injection pain drawing and numeric pain scale.

The same procedure was repeated at the L4 and L3 nerve levels at one-week intervals. Each time the patient filled out a pre- and post-injection pain assessment.

The patient had 90% pain relief after the L5 selective nerve root injection (Fig. 2.1) and no pain relief after the L4 and L3 nerve injections (Fig. 2.2).

Any pain relief over 80% would have been considered a positive diagnostic injection.[9] The patient was given a copy of the three pre- and post-injection pain diagrams for the surgeon. The diagnostic selective nerve injections were useful in diagnosing an atypical L5 radiculopathy (Fig. 2.3). The surgeon was confident in the responses of the diagnostic injections and went on to perform an anterior and posterior L5-S1 interbody fusion. Postoperatively, the patient had 90% relief of his symptoms and resumed his previous functional level.

It is important to note that while the diagnostic injections can more accurately pinpoint the pain generator when conventional methods fail, they cannot predict surgical outcomes. Additionally, false positives can occur if the procedure is not carried out correctly. Improper spread of the anesthetic to other nerve root levels or around the sinuvertebral nerve can anesthetize nontargeted potential pain generators.[10] A proper contrast dye flow pattern and small volume of anesthetic (less than half a milliliter) can reduce some of these concerns.[11]

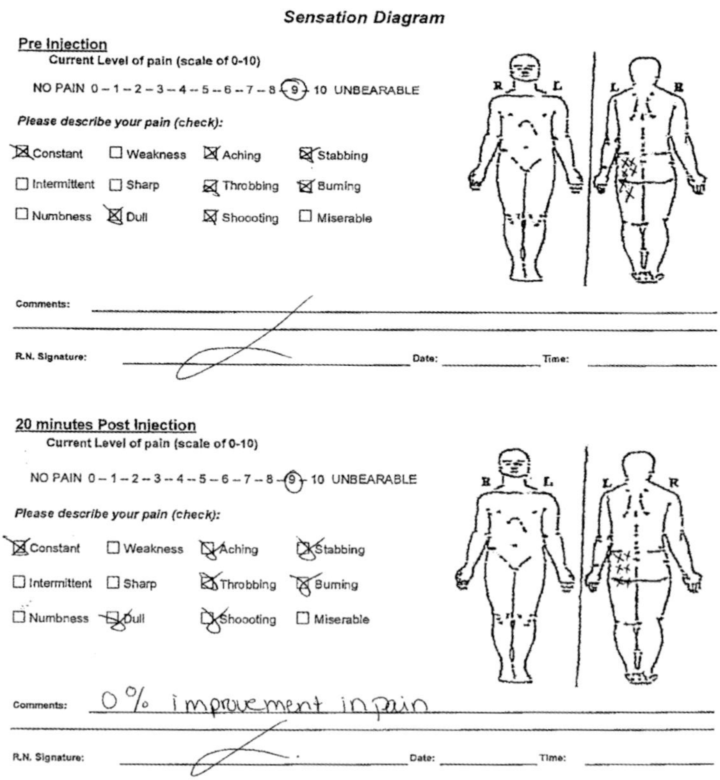

Sensation Diagram

Pre Injection

Current Level of pain (scale of 0-10)

NO PAIN 0 – 1 – 2 – 3 – 4 – 5 – 6 – 7 – 8 – (9) – 10 UNBEARABLE

Please describe your pain (check):

[X] Constant [ ] Weakness [X] Aching [X] Stabbing

[ ] Intermittent [ ] Sharp [X] Throbbing [X] Burning

[ ] Numbness [X] Dull [X] Shooting [ ] Miserable

Comments:

R.N. Signature: Date: Time:

20 minutes Post Injection

Current Level of pain (scale of 0-10)

NO PAIN 0 – 1 – 2 – 3 – 4 – 5 – 6 – 7 – 8 – (9) – 10 UNBEARABLE

Please describe your pain (check):

[X] Constant [ ] Weakness [X] Aching [X] Stabbing

[ ] Intermittent [ ] Sharp [X] Throbbing [X] Burning

[ ] Numbness [X] Dull [X] Shooting [ ] Miserable

Comments: 0% improvement in pain

R.N. Signature: Date: Time:

Fig. 2.2: Pain diagram pre-selective spinal nerve injection and post-selective spinal nerve injection performed for the left L3 and L4 spinal nerves. Note that the patient reports 0% relief of his typical pain

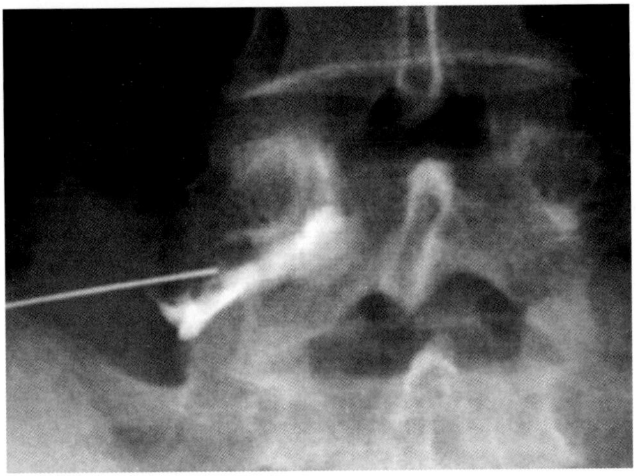

Fig. 2.3: Left L5 selective spinal nerve injection. Note the contrast along the spinal nerve, but not extending past the medial border of the L5 pedicle

SUMMARY

Selective nerve root injections can be a useful tool for diagnosing an atypical presentation of radicular pain. The indication for such a procedure includes an atypical radicular pattern with equivocal findings on physical examination and diagnostic studies. This intervention should be considered only when the resulting diagnostic information would impact the treatment intervention.

REFERENCES

1. Dillingham TR. Electrodiagnostic approach to patients with suspected radiculopathy. Physical Medicine and Rehabilitation Clinics of North America. 2002;13:567-88.
2. Berg S, Isberg B, Josephson A, et al. The impact of discography on the surgical decision in patients with chronic low back pain. The Spine Journal: Official Journal of the North American Spine Society. 2012;12:283-91.
3. Carragee EJ, Lincoln T, Parmar VS, et al. A gold standard evaluation of the "discogenic pain" diagnosis as determined by provocative discography. Spine. 2006;31:2115-23.
4. Carragee EJ, Don AS, Hurwitz EL, et al. 2009 ISSLS Prize Winner: Does discography cause accelerated progression of degeneration changes in the lumbar disc: a ten-year matched cohort study. Spine. 2009;34:2338-45.
5. Krempen JF, Smith BS. Nerve-root injection: a method for evaluating the etiology of sciatica. The Journal of Bone and Joint Surgery American volume. 1974;56:1435-44.
6. Huston CW, Slipman CW. Diagnostic selective nerve root blocks: indications and usefulness. Physical Medicine and Rehabilitation Clinics of North America. 2002;13:545-65.

7. Slipman CW, Issac Z. The role of diagnostic selective nerve root blocks in the management of spinal pain. Pain Physician. 2001;4:214-26.
8. Bogduk N, Aprill CN, Derby R. Epidural spinal injections. St. Louis: Mosby; 1995.
9. Derby R, Kine G, Saal JA, et al. Response to steroid and duration of radicular pain as predictors of surgical outcome. Spine. 1992;17:S176-83.
10. Bogduk N, Tynan W, Wilson AS. The nerve supply to the human lumbar intervertebral discs. Journal of Anatomy. 1981;132:39-56.
11. Furman MB, Lee TS, Mehta A, et al. Contrast flow selectivity during transforaminal lumbosacral epidural steroid injections. Pain Physician. 2008; 11:855-61.

3 Lumbar Disc Herniation with Radiculopathy: Lumbar Transforaminal Epidural Steroid Injection

Natacha Falcon, Jeremy Simon

CHIEF COMPLAINT

The patient complains about low back pain with left leg pain.

HISTORY OF PRESENT ILLNESS

This patient is a 32-year-old right-handed male with a history of lower back pain for 2 years. He has a history of an L5-S1 microdiscectomy 6 months ago for recalcitrant low back and left lower extremity pain. The pain reoccurred 1 month ago while lifting a heavy piece of equipment at work. After the event, he began experiencing lower back pain with radiation into the left lower extremity. He rated the back pain as 4/10, and the left radicular symptoms as an 8/10. He describes the pain as an achy and sharp pain in the lower lumbar area with a burning pain into the posterior lateral aspect of his thigh and leg. The pain is constant and aggravated by sitting, bending and twisting. Standing and changing positions frequently help reduce his pain. The pain is similar to the pain he experienced previously prior to his surgery.

The patient has had an epidural steroid injection with transient relief of his pain prior to his left L5-S1 microdiscectomy. The surgery did provide the patient with resolution of his symptoms, until the above mentioned work injury.

He denies any weakness, bowel or bladder incontinence. He takes anti-inflammatories occasionally with mild pain relief. He attended physical therapy for 2 weeks without relief of his symptoms.

REVIEW OF SYSTEMS

Denies

PAST MEDICAL HISTORY

The patient denies any past medical history.

SURGICAL HISTORY

Left L5-S1 microdiscectomy 6 months prior.

MEDICATIONS

Ibuprofen

ALLERGIES

No known drug allergies.

FAMILY HISTORY

Noncontributory

SOCIAL HISTORY

Alcohol socially, no tobacco, or drug use. He works in construction but admits he does not follow his lifting restrictions as outlined after surgery.

The pain diagram of the patient is shown in Figure 3.1.

PHYSICAL EXAMINATION

General: Pleasant, cooperative, alert and oriented, no acute distress.

Inspection: No asymmetry, no evidence of scoliosis, well-healed scar consistent with prior lumbar surgery.

Gait: Non-antalgic, able to ambulate on heels, toes and tandem without difficulty.

Range of Motion: *Limitations in flexion with more pain reproduction in flexion than extension.*

Neurological:

- *Strength*: Manual muscle testing 5/5 with exception of left dorsiflexion and *extensor hallucis longus 4/5*
- *Sensation*: Decreased light touch and pinprick over dorsum of foot on the left
- *Reflexes*: Symmetrical bilateral patellae and Achilles reflex
- *Provocative*: Straight leg raise and sitting dural tension signs—negative.

Musculoskeletal: Hip internal and external with pain free normal range of motion, FABER (Flexion, abduction, external rotation) test: negative bilaterally.

Pain Diagram

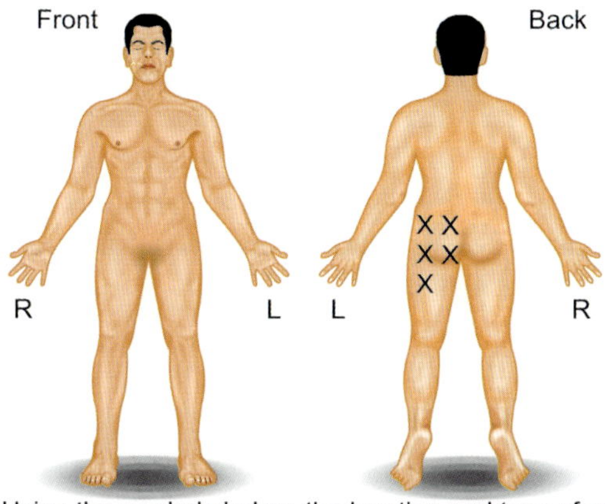

Using the symbols below, the location and type of pain sensations are marked on the diagrams. All the affected areas are included.

TYPE OF SENSATIONS

Aching	^ ^ ^ ^ ^ ^
Sharp or stabbing	X X X X X X
Burning	//////////
Pins and needles	--------------
Numbness	0 0 0 0 0 0

Fig. 3.1: Pain diagram

IMAGING

Lumbar spine X-rays: Normal segmentation. No scoliosis. No evidence for fractures or spondylolisthesis. There is evidence of a prior laminotomy on the left at L5-S1. Reduced disc space height is noted at L5-S1.

Lumbar spine MRI with and without Gadolinium: Recurrent left paracentral disc herniation at L5-S1. Loss of lumbar lordosis is noted, likely secondary to muscle spasms. Moderate degenerative disc disease at L5-S1 and interval left L5-S1 hemilaminectomy. Postcontrast images show enhancing scar and granulation tissue at the left paraspinal region without abnormal fluid collection.

DIAGNOSIS

Lumbar radiculopathy; Left L5-S1; secondary to recurrent left paracentral disc herniation.

NONINTERVENTIONAL TREATMENT OPTIONS

Conservative management of radicular pain begins with activity modifications and physical therapy. The focus of physical therapy is improvement in functional abilities, centralization of pain, body mechanics education, and instruction in individualized home exercise program (HEP). Physical therapy that emphasizes the McKenzie approach has been shown to aid in centralization of pain.[1,2] Centralization of pain refers to movement of the pain from the leg or buttock and into the low back.[1] Modalities such as ice, heat, ultrasound and transcutaneous electrical stimulation (TENS) may provide additional analgesic benefits as well.[3,4] Physical therapy aids in return to function and minimizes the sequela of immobility.

Medication management is used to decrease acute pain, so patients may better able return to function. Oral corticosteroids are often prescribed for radicular pain, although there is a lack of evidence supporting its use in this condition.[5] Nonsteroidal anti-inflammatory drugs (NSAIDs) are effective for short-term symptomatic relief in patients with acute low back pain.[6] Muscle relaxants may be used acutely for spasms and pain. Non-narcotic and narcotic pain medications may be utilized if the patient is not responsive to physical therapy and NSAIDs alone, or should the patient have a contraindication to taking NSAIDs. Neuropathic agents such as gabapentin and pregabalin may be utilized as well for radicular pain. These agents presumably work by binding to the voltage-gated calcium channels and may serve to "stabilize" hyperexcitable axons.[7] Some antidepressant medications, such as tricyclic antidepressants, have been shown to be efficacious with neuropathic pain as well and are believed to work by increasing the amount of norepinephrine and serotonin in the presynaptic membrane, as well as other proposed mechanisms.[7,8]

INTERVENTIONAL OPTIONS

Lumbar Transforaminal Epidural Steroid Injection (LTFESI)

Lumbar radicular pain (sciatica) is defined as pain referred from the back into the dermatome of the affected nerve root along the femoral or sciatic nerve trunk. Radiculitis implies there are no neurological deficits; radiculopathy implies there are neurological deficits such as motor or sensory abnormalities.

In the absence of neurologic deficits (progressive weakness, bowel or bladder incontinence) and failure of conservative measures (physical therapy and medication management) consideration of an epidural steroid injection is appropriate. Thus far, evidence is conflicting regarding the efficacy of epidural steroid injections. In clinical practice, many patients find relief in epidural steroid injections. There is no one single intervention that will help all patients with radicular pain. Time since onset of symptoms is one prognostic indicator of success with epidural steroid injections. Some data indicates that patients with acute radicular pain (less than 3 months) respond better to transforaminal injections than those with radicular symptoms greater than one year.[9]

Transforaminal injections have been shown to be efficacious for lumbar radicular pain and may potentially eliminate the need for surgery.[10] A combination of physical therapy and epidural steroid injections are usually effective for patients with herniated nucleus propulsus (HNP) to avoid surgery, as indicated in trial of Riew et al.[10]

Potential complications of lumbar transforaminal epidural steroid injections have been reported.[11-14] The use of fluoroscopy with live injection of contrast significantly reduces the risk of vascular injection.[15] Utilization of digital subtraction angiography, while not available on all fluoroscopy units, may add additional safety in identifying vascular flow. A case report showed a resultant paraplegia with a right L5 transforaminal epidural steroid injection with triamcinolone despite digital subtraction, however.[16] Paraplegia most commonly results from embolization of a particulate steroid into a vessel that communicates with the spinal cord.[14]

PATIENT DISCUSSION

The patient has a past medical history significant for a previous left L5-S1 microdiscectomy with complete resolution of his symptoms. He had surgical intervention following failed conservative measures of physical therapy, medication management, and an epidural steroid injection.

The patient now has a return of his symptoms with magnetic resonance imaging (MRI) evidence of a recurrent disc herniation.

PLAN

Patient's pain pattern is in the L5-S1 dermatomal distribution. He has motor weakness in his left dorsiflexion (L4-5) and left extensor hallucis longus (L5). He has sensory changes over the dorsum of his left foot (L5). He has MRI evidence of a recurrent left paracentral disc herniation at L5-S1. It is minimally contacting the left S1 nerve root and is causing significant lateral recess narrowing. There is also moderate left neural foraminal narrowing, thus explaining the patient's L5 pattern of involvement. Given his history, physical examination findings, and MRI results, a left L5-S1 transforaminal epidural steroid injection (TFESI) was ordered (Fig. 3.2).

A S1 TFESI could have been considered as well, as a paracentral disc herniation will likely affect the traversing S1 nerve root, and a far lateral disc herniation would likely affect the L5 spinal nerve. Due to the patient's

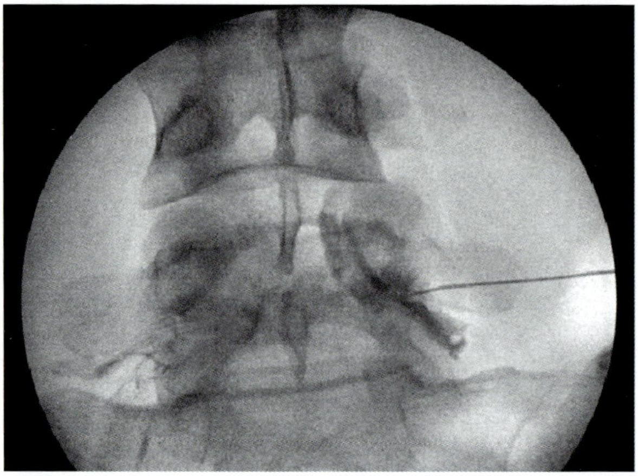

Fig. 3.2: Left L5 transforaminal epidural steroid injection. Note the flow of contrast extending medial to the pedicle and extending to the L4-L5 disc space

presentation in the L5 dermatomal distribution, a second level was not deemed necessary.

Left L5-S1 Transforaminal Epidural Steroid Injection

The risks, benefits and alternatives of the procedure were discussed extensively with the patient. Risks discussed included but were not limited to bleeding, infection, allergic reaction and structural damage. Written informed consent was obtained from the patient and then the following procedure was performed.

The patient was placed in the prone position on the fluoroscopy table. The C-arm was rotated to a slightly oblique and ipsilateral position. The lumbar area was prepped and draped in the usual sterile fashion. Next, the left L5-S1 neuroforamen was identified under fluoroscopic guidance. Using sterile technique, the superficial skin was anesthetized with 1% Lidocaine (preservative-free) using a 25-gauge, 1½-inch needle. Next, a sterile 22-gauge (5-inch) spinal needle was advanced down to the 6 o'clock area of the pedicle under intermittent fluoroscopic guidance, targeting the superior, lateral aspect of the "safe triangle". Multiplanar fluoroscopic imaging was used to further verify needle placement. One cc of Omnipaque-240 contrast was injected through microbore tubing under live fluoroscopy. There was no intravascular uptake observed. There was a medial and superior epidural flow pattern observed. After aspiration was negative for return of blood or cerebrospinal fluid, a solution of 2 mL of Kenalog (40 mg/mL) and 2 cc of 1% Lidocaine (preservative-free) was injected into the left neuroforamen at the L5-S1 level.

The needle was then removed. No blood or cerebrospinal fluid (CSF) was noted to be draining, and a sterile band-aid was applied after pressure was applied with a gauze pad. Pulse oximetry was used throughout the procedure and the patient's pulse and oxygen saturation remained within normal limits. Vital signs remained normal and were monitored for an additional 20 minutes. The patient tolerated the procedure well. There were no complications noted and no new neurological complaints.

The patient was instructed to apply local ice over the injected site for 10–15 minutes for the next 24–48 hours. The patient was instructed by the authors to contact them if there are any problems. A postprocedure instruction sheet was given.

Fluoroscopy was utilized to ascertain that the needle was placed as close as possible to the source of pathology, and that the injectate was not injected into a blood vessel or into the thecal sac.

Anterior-posterior, oblique and lateral views were checked and it was ascertained that the Omnipaque is in the epidural space at the L5-S1 level on the left side. Pictures were taken to document accurate placement of the medication (*see* Fig. 3.2).

At the patient's follow-up visit, 2 weeks after the left L5-S1 TFESI, he had marked improvement in his low back and lower extremity pain. His pain scores had improved to 4/10 in his lower back and 1/10 in his lower extremity.

REFERENCES

1. Wheeler AH. Diagnosis and management of low back pain and sciatica. American Family Physician. 1995;52:1333-41, 1347-8.
2. Taylor MD. The McKenzie method: a general practice interpretation: the lumbar spine. Australian Family Physician. 1996;25:189-93, 196-7, 200-1.
3. Brosseau L, Milne S, Robinson V, et al. Efficacy of the transcutaneous electrical nerve stimulation for the treatment of chronic low back pain: a meta-analysis. Spine. 2002;27:596-603.
4. Milne S, Welch V, Brosseau L, et al. Transcutaneous electrical nerve stimulation (TENS) for chronic low back pain. Cochrane database of systematic reviews 2001:CD003008.
5. Haimovic IC, Beresford HR. Dexamethasone is not superior to placebo for treating lumbosacral radicular pain. Neurology. 1986;36:1593-4.
6. van Tulder MW, Scholten RJ, Koes BW, et al. Non-steroidal anti-inflammatory drugs for low back pain. Cochrane database of systematic reviews 2000:CD000396.
7. Lipetz JS, Malanga GA. Oral medications in the treatment of acute low back pain. Occup Med. 1998;13:151-66.
8. Staiger TO, Gaster B, Sullivan MD, et al. Systematic review of antidepressants in the treatment of chronic low back pain. Spine. 2003;28:2540-5.
9. Slipman CW, Derby R, Simeone FA, et al. Interventional spine: an algorithmic approach. Philadelphia, PA: Elsevier; 2008.

10. Riew KD, Yin Y, Gilula L, et al. The effect of nerve-root injections on the need for operative treatment of lumbar radicular pain: a prospective, randomized, controlled, double-blind study. The Journal of Bone and Joint Surgery, American volume. 2000;82-A:1589-93.
11. Krause D, Guiu B, Lerais J-M, et al. Lumbar transforaminal epidural injections: evaluation of potential risks and complications. Journal de radiologie. 2010; 91:1086-92.
12. Karaman H, Kavak GO, Tufek A, et al. The complications of transforaminal lumbar epidural steroid injections. Spine. 2011;36:E819-24.
13. Goodman BS, Posecion LW, Mallempati S, et al. Complications and pitfalls of lumbar interlaminar and transforaminal epidural injections. Current Reviews in Musculoskeletal Medicine. 2008;1:212-22.
14. Kennedy DJ, Dreyfuss P, Aprill CN,et al. Paraplegia following image-guided transforaminal lumbar spine epidural steroid injection: two case reports. Pain Medicine. 2009;10:1389-94.
15. Furman MB, O'Brien EM, Zgleszewski TM. Incidence of intravascular penetration in transforaminal lumbosacral epidural steroid injections. Spine. 2000;25:2628-32.
16. Chang Chien GC, Candido KD, Knezevic NN. Digital subtraction angiography does not reliably prevent paraplegia associated with lumbar transforaminal epidural steroid injection. Pain Physician. 2012;15:515-23.

4

Lumbar Spinal Stenosis with Radiculopathy

Michael Molter, Jeremy Simon

CHIEF COMPLAINT

The patient complains about low back pain and pain in both legs.

HISTORY OF PRESENT ILLNESS

The patient is a pleasant 57-year-old male with low back and bilateral lower extremity pain. The symptoms have been present over the last 6 months. The axial component is located in the lower lumbar spine and is described as a constant ache. There are times when it becomes sharp in nature primarily with moving from a bent position to an erect posture. It radiates across the lower back region. These symptoms are associated with paresthesias and pain in the bilateral lower extremities. Both legs affected equally. The leg pain is constant, located over the anterior thigh to the dorsal aspect of his feet (Fig. 4.1—Pain diagram). He rates the pain level at 7/10 on a numeric scale today and is anywhere from 5–9/10 on average. His back pain and leg pain are equal in regards to their severity and how they affect his regular activities. Sitting is the only thing that has helped his symptoms. His symptoms are worse with walking and standing for extended periods of time. Furthermore, he feels unstable when he has to ambulate any significant distance secondary to the pain in his legs. He denies any associated bowel or bladder incontinence/retention, fever, chills, night sweats, unintentional weight loss, progressive weakness or saddle type anesthesia. The pain does not waken him at night, but he is often sleeping in a reclining chair due to pain with lying in bed. He has had no treatments in regards to therapy, injections, or medications at this time.

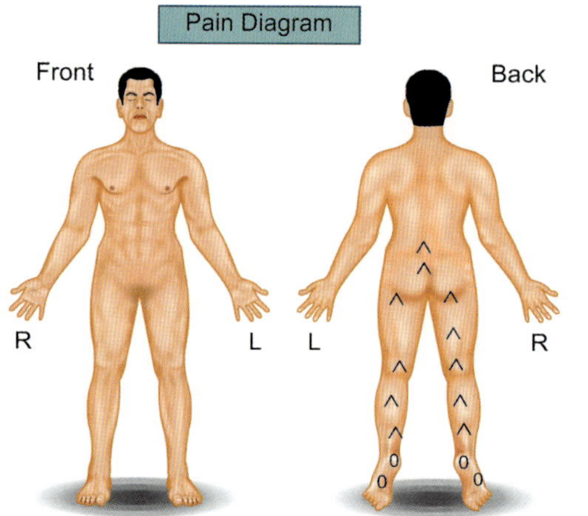

Using the symbols below, the location and type of pain sensations are marked on the diagrams. All the affected areas are included.

TYPE OF SENSATIONS

Aching	^ ^ ^ ^ ^ ^
Sharp or stabbing	X X X X X X
Burning	//////////
Pins and needles	---------------
Numbness	0 0 0 0 0 0

Fig. 4.1: Pain diagram

PAST MEDICAL HISTORY

Significant for a history of a deep vein thrombosis (DVT), since resolved, hypertension, osteoarthritis and venous insufficiency.

PAST SURGICAL HISTORY

None

REVIEW OF SYSTEMS

Positive for low back pain as well as bilateral leg pain. Positive for hypertension, osteoarthritis, as well as swelling in the lower extremities, DVT and reflux disease.

FAMILY HISTORY

Diabetes mellitus

SOCIAL HISTORY

A 40-pack-year of tobacco use. He works as an engineering technician in Navy yard, prior to that he worked directly in building at the Navy yard. He is married. Ambulation is limited secondary to pain in his legs. He is only able to ambulate a half of a block without pain in both legs.

MEDICATIONS

Coumadin, Norvasc, Zestril, Antivert and Omeprazole.

ALLERGIES

Ibuprofen sensitivity, when taken causes him severe vomiting.

PHYSICAL EXAMINATION

A 57-year-old male who appears his stated age, in no apparent distress.

Vital signs: blood pressure: 132/90 mm Hg, pulse: 80/min, height: 6 feet 4 inches, weight: 225 lbs, body mass index (BMI): 27.4.

Cardiovascular examination: Distal pulses intact in the lower extremities at 2/4 bilaterally. Nonpitting edema to level of ankle bilaterally. No calf pain is noted bilaterally.

Musculoskeletal evaluation: His lower extremity range of motion is normal in the knee and hip joints. No pain with range of motion testing in bilateral knee or hip joints. No piriformis muscle, sacroiliac joint or greater trochanteric tenderness to palpation is noted. *He has paraspinal tenderness noted in the right and left side*. No spinous process tenderness is noted. No lumbar paraspinal spasms are noted. His lumbar spine range of motion demonstrates flexion to be normal and without pain. *He has decreased extension to 10 degrees secondary to pain in lumbar spine*. Negative straight leg, slump, Patrick's and Gaenslen's test bilaterally.

His neurologic examination demonstrates his reflexes to be *1+/4 bilaterally in the lower extremities*. There are no cerebellar signs noted. Manual muscle testing in the bilateral hip flexors, hip extensors, tibialis anterior, extensor hallucis longus (EHL) and gastrocsoleus is 5/5 bilaterally. He is oriented to person, place and time. Normal muscle bulk and tone for age. Sensation is intact to light touch, pinprick and proprioception in the bilateral lower extremity dermatomes. Babinski reveals downgoing toes and Hoffman's sign is negative bilaterally.

X-rays lumbar spine: Anterior/posterior, flexion and extension X-rays of the lumbar spine demonstrate normal segmentation, no significant scoliosis, and *mild degenerative changes noted at the L3-L4, L4-L5, and L5-S1 level without spondylolysis or spondylolisthesis*. There is no instability on flexion/extension views.

Magnetic resonance imaging (MRI) lumbar spine: *Multilevel lumbar spondylosis central disc protrusion at L3-L4 as well as moderate central stenosis at L4-L5 and L5-S1 levels*. No significant neuroforaminal narrowing is appreciated. No spondylolisthesis or spondylolysis noted.

DIAGNOSIS

Lumbar spinal stenosis with bilateral radiculopathy, L4-L5.

Discussion

His symptoms are consistent with L4 and L5 radiculopathy as the L4 and L5 dermatomes are affected. There is also associated lower back pain, decreased lumbar spine range of motion, particularly with extension.

The word "stenosis" is derived from Greek and means "narrow". The prevalence of lumbar stenosis is estimated to be 2.45 million older men and 3.54 million older women who have symptoms suggestive of central/lumbar stenosis according to data from the 2000 census.[1]

This entity remains the number one preoperative diagnosis for adults older than 65 years to have lumbar spine surgery.[2] A long-term study of lumbar stenosis patients has noted of patients followed 70% were unchanged, 15% improved, 15% worsened.[3]

Classification of lumbar stenosis is divided into congenital/developmental which includes idiopathic and achondroplastic. The acquired type includes degenerative (most common), combination of degenerative and congenital, spondylytic/spondylolisthesthetic, iatrogenic, post-traumatic, and metabolic.[4] Kirkaldy-Willis described the pathophysiology involving a three joint complex of zygapophysial joints and the intervertebral disc. This process leads to dysfunction, instability and finally stability of vertebral column. Through a cascade of events, rotation and compression injuries cause degenerative changes of the described three joint complex. The end result is degeneration/loss of height of the intervertebral disc, hypertrophy of the ligamentum flavum, and overgrowth of the lumbar zygapophysial joints, leading to narrowing in the spinal canal.[5]

Lumbar spinal stenosis typically can involve lateral or central locations. Central stenosis is found at the intervertebral level caused by multitude of factors including ligamentum flavum hypertrophy or buckling, disc protrusion, hypertrophic zygapophysial joints and degenerative spondylolisthesis. Patients with central stenosis typically present with neurogenic claudication symptoms.[6] Lateral stenosis symptomatology results from compression within the lateral recess area which is medial to pedicle, the midzone located under the pars interarticularis and pedicle, and the exit zone/neuroforaminal region.[6] Hypertrophy of any of the structures can result in radicular symptoms. It is believed that the radiating pain in the lower extremities is caused by neural ischemia from compression of the vasa nervorum, myelin sheath and axons or venous congestion.[7]

Patients with lumbar spinal stenosis present with neurogenic claudication, increasing bilateral leg pain and paresthesias that are exacerbated with prolonged standing and ambulation, and typically resolved by rest. Flexion typically alleviates the patients' symptomatology, where extension, walking downhill can flare up the symptoms of patients.[8]

TREATMENT OPTIONS

Smoking cessation: With the patient's noted 40-pack-year history of tobacco use, he is at risk of increased degenerative changes as well as decreased amount of blood flow and subsequent nutrition to the intervertebral disc.[9]

Weight loss: According to CDC specifications, the patient's BMI of 27.4 puts him in the overweight category.[10] Being overweight is associated with increased risk of low back pain.[11] It is shown that spine mobility and disc nutrition decreases with increased body weight.[12] This also leads to an increase in compressive force throughout the spine during regular activities.[13] A recommendation should be made to seek a nutritional evaluation for further dietary alterations to alleviate increased axial loading secondary to his increased body weight.

Due to multiple comorbidities, he was not a candidate for nonsteroidal anti-inflammatory use. His chronic anticoagulant use in combination with a nonsteroidals would put him at increased risk of bleeding secondary to antiplatelet effect as well as gastric mucosal damage.[14] Those older than 65 years of age, where patients taking both warfarin and nonsteroidals, had a thirteen fold risk in hemorrhagic peptic ulcers than those taking either drug.[15] He did not have an interest in other pain medications due to intolerance of opiates and muscle relaxers. Considerations for him could include possible use of membrane stabilizing agent to help with some of his radicular pain. One option for this may include gabapentin which acts to decrease pain by modifying the excitability of nerve or muscle through effects of sodium and calcium channels or by promoting the inhibition of gamma-aminobutyric acid alpha (GABA-α) receptors.[16,17] There has been an increased incidence of lower extremity edema compared to placebo in studies of patients taking gabapentin.[18]

Physical therapy: Physical therapy program in this case should be designed to introduce mechanical changes to lumbar spine to open up neurovascular space through increased flexion as well as restoring intervertebral motion of lumbar segments.[19] Progression to a full flexion based program is tied to first improving and restoring intersegmental motion. This can involve using intervertebral glides and distraction techniques.[20] The use of education, awareness and exercises can aid in decreasing compressive loading forces on the spine and improving posture.[21] Finally, a general conditioning program is essentially to long-term maintenance and improvement in conditioning.[22] Recommendations are usually for a program two times a week for 4 weeks with re-assessment by the physician at that time. After 4 weeks of physical therapy, the patient noted some improvement in his lumbar spinal range of motion and a slight improvement in his lower back pain. He also noted doing a home exercise program on a daily basis as well. His leg symptoms continued despite this intervention.

It was then decided to proceed with an L4-5 interlaminar epidural steroid injection with the hope of reducing the patient's pain and improving his overall function. This level and approach was chosen secondary to the fact that patient's noted symptomatology corresponded with the L4 and L5 dermatomes and stenosis noted primarily in a central location.

Lumbar Interlaminar Injections

Indications: Studies are conflicting in the effectiveness of lumbar interlaminar epidural steroid infections.[40]

- Lumbar spinal stenosis
- Lumbar neuroforaminal stenosis[23]

Interlaminar injections are based on approach to dorsal epidural space by placing a needle between the laminae. The epidural space surrounds the thecal sac and is bounded by the posterior longitudinal ligament anteriorly, ligamentum flavum and periosteum of laminae posteriorly and the pedicles of spinal column and intervertebral foramina containing their elements laterally.[24]

Level injected: L4-L5 paramedian approach using a 20-gauge, 3 ½-inch Tuohy needle.

The procedure was performed in block suite with fluoroscopic guidance. Risks and benefits of the procedure were discussed with the patient. Consent of the patient was obtained and the following procedure was performed.

The patient was placed in the prone position on the fluoroscopic table. The back was prepped with Betadine and draped in the usual sterile fashion. The lumbar spine was visualized in anterior-posterior (AP) view. The L4-L5 interlaminar space was identified. The skin insertion site was anesthetized with a combination of 3 cc 1% Xylocaine and 1 cc bicarbonate using a 25-gauge, 1½-inch needle. Using a 20-gauge, 3½-inch Tuohy was inserted via a paramedian

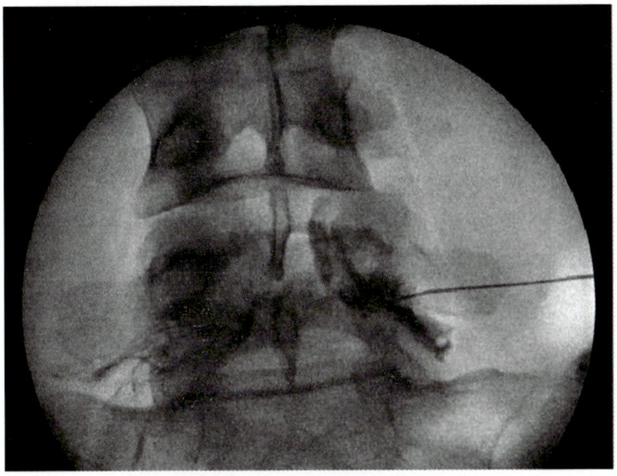

Fig. 4.2: A posterior-anterior image of a right paramedian L5-S1 interlaminar epidural steroid injection

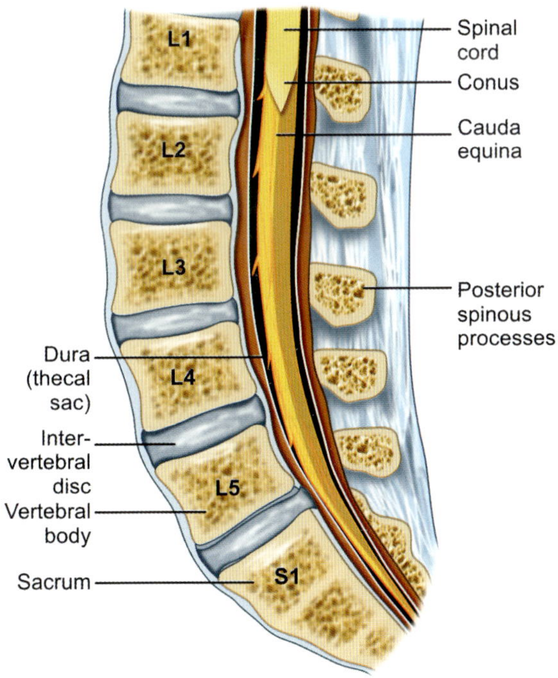

Fig. 4.3: A lateral image of an L5-S1 interlaminar epidural steroid injection. Note the needle at the spinolaminar line and the flow of contrast appearing as a straight line (bound by the ligamentum flavum posteriorly and the thecal sac anteriorly) indicating epidural placement

approach. The needle was directed in a bull's eye approach until it contacted the inferior lamina. The lumbar spine was visualized in AP and lateral views (Figs 4.2 and 4.3). The needle was then redirected cephalad and medial. The needle was advanced into the ligamentum flavum (Fig. 4.4). A loss of

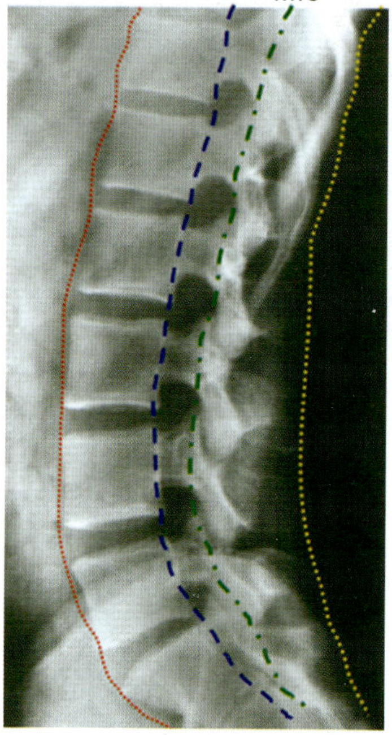

Fig. 4.4: Spinolaminar line

resistance to normal saline technique was then used. There was good frank loss of resistance. There was no cerebrospinal fluid (CSF) or heme aspirated. There were no paresthesias.

Two milliliters of Omnipaque 240 was injected under live fluoroscopy and flow of contrast was noted. There was good epidural spread (*see* Fig. 4.3). There was no intrathecal or intravascular uptake. Therapeutic injection consisted of 3 ml preservative-free sodium chloride and 1 cc of 6 mg/cc betametha sone.

The needle was flushed and removed intact. The patient was taken to recovery in stable condition.

COMPLICATIONS/PITFALLS

Dural punctures have a rate of approximately 0.5–5%.[25] This occurs secondary to the needle passing beyond into the spinal space. Variables affecting this can be severity of stenosis with possible adherence of layers or redundancy of the ligamentum flavum. Increased risk factors include women during pregnancy, low BMI, age between 18 years and 30 years with declines in percentage in children younger than age 13 and adults older than 60 years of age.[26] Symptoms may include positional headaches, most notably worse when going from a laying to standing or a seated position. The headache can be quite severe, dull, nonthrobbing and fronto-occipital in nature.[27] Initial treatment includes having the patient increase their fluid intake.[28] Caffeine may also be utilized. Should symptoms fail to improve, consideration may be given to an autologous blood patch. This involves drawing a patient's blood and injecting it into epidural space to seal the area of puncture. Epidural blood patch remains the invasive of treatment of choice with success rates of approximately 70% after initial injection.[28,29] In trying to prevent a dural puncture, the physician may consider use of smaller gauge, noncutting needles as well as using lateral views on X-ray to check for depth of needle placement.[28]

Subarachnoid Injection

Occurs due to improper depth of needle and penetration of the subarachnoid space. The resultant symptoms are secondary to the amount of anesthetic directly injected.[30] Symptoms associated with this included disorientation, lightheadedness, complete motor and sensory block, respiratory depression and seizures.[30] If a high spinal were to occur, fluid resuscitation for hypotension and maintaining the airway are of paramount importance. IV access should be obtained prior to the procedure and a certification by the interventional physician should be obtained in cardiopulmonary resuscitation and advanced cardiac life support. A crash cart should be available and medications/equipment periodically checked for expiration and function. Use of lateral view to assess depth as well as assessment of the contrast pattern.[24]

Epidural Abscess

Typically a rare complication with a single shot epidural injection.[31] Symptoms include back pain, fever, chills, progressive weakness in lower extremities, etc.[24] Labs may demonstrate an elevated white blood cell count. Imaging may demonstrate increased enhancement in area of the epidural space. Treatment involves hospitalization, appropriate antibiotics as well as surgical evaluation. Preventative aspects include use of a sterile technique, using single-use vials, as well as appropriate skin prep.

Epidural Hematoma

This complication is an expansion of blood compressing the epidural region and structures of the spinal canal. It has been reported to occur in less than 1:150,000 patients.[32] Epidural hematomas are rare in patients with normal clotting factors. The presentation is often progressive neurologic dysfunction in the lower extremities as well as possible cauda equina syndrome.[33] Magnetic resonance imaging typically demonstrates an expanding space compressing lesion. Treatment involves emergent laminectomy for decompression of the lesion. It is imperative to have patients evaluated if a hematoma is suspected as surgical outcome is improved with quicker surgical decompression.[34] Preventing this complication includes close monitoring of high-risk patients both pre- and post-procedure. Preprocedure lab work should be done on those patients with platelets needing to be greater than 100,000 and International Normalized Ratio (INR), not prothrombin time, less than 1.2-1.5, depending on the reference[35] prothrombin time (PT) less than 1.2. Furthermore, communication with the prescribing physician on blood thinners in regards to high-risk patient and risk benefit ratio on a case-by-case basis. They must always be consulted in regards to the holding of anticoagulants.[35]

Intravascular Injection

Intravascular injection is more common with needle placement in the lateral portion of the spinal canal than midline due to the dorsolateral location of the vertebral venous plexus.[24,36] Intravascular uptake in lumbar epidural steroid injections can be up to 1.9%.[37] Severity of symptoms is usually dose dependent in the absence of allergic reaction.[38] Symptoms range from dizziness, tinnitus, and disorientation to seizures, unconsciousness and coma.[24] Treatment remains supportive in these cases. Preventions include injection of nonionic contrast with use of live fluoroscopy as well as digital subtraction, if available.[24]

Anatomical

Bony landmarks include both the superficial and deep oss. The superficial oss that may be encountered is the spinous process. Deep oss is consistent with the lamina proper. If proper technique is used with fluoroscopy, contact of spinous process should be limited. It is possible to get a false loss of resistance secondary to adipose and connective tissues. One method of differentiating between soft tissue and epidural space is to inject saline with a small air bubble in the syringe. Saline in the epidural space will not compress the bubble, but if it is in soft tissue it will compress.[39] Use of lateral X-ray for depth guidance can also assist in this matter.

REFERENCES

1. Vogt MT, Cawthorn PM, Kang JD, et al. Prevalence of symptoms of cervical and lumbar stenosis among participants in the osteoporotic fractures in men study. Spine. 2006;31(13):1445-51.
2. Katz J, Harris M. Lumbar spinal stenosis. The New England Journal of Medicine. 2008;358(8):818-25.

3. Johnsson KE, Rosen I, Udeu A. The natural course of lumbar spinal stenosis. Clin Orthop Relat Res. 1992;(279):82-6.
4. Arnoldi CC, Brodshy AE, Cauchoix J. Lumbar spinal stenosis and nerve root entrapments: definition and classification. Clinic Orthop. 1976; 115:4-5.
5. Kirkaldy-Willis WH, Wedge JH, Yong-Hing K, et al. Pathology and pathogenesis of lumbar spondylosis and stenosis. Spine.1978;3:319-28.
6. Botwin KP, Gruber RD. Lumbar spinal stenosis: anatomy and pathogenesis. Physical Medicine Rehabilitation Clinics of North America. 2003; 14(1):1-15.
7. Rydevik B, Brown MD, Lundberg G. Pathoanatomy and pathophysiology of nerve root compression. Spine. 1984;9(1):7-15.
8. Barr KP, Harrast MA. Low back pain. In: Braddom R (Ed). Physical Medicine and Rehabilitation. 3rd edition. Philadelphia: Elsevier; 2007.pp.918-9.
9. Porter SE, Hanley EN Jr. The musculoskeletal effects of smoking. J Am Acad Orthop Surg. 2001;9(1):9-17.
10. Maggard-Gibbons M, Maglione M, Livhits M, et al. Bariatric surgery for weight loss and glycemic control in nonmorbidly obese adults with diabetes: a systematic review. JAMA, 2013;309(21):2250-61.
11. Rahman Shiri, Karppinen Jaro, Leino-Arjas Paivi, et al. The association between obesity and low back pain: a meta analysis. American Journal of Epidemiology. 2010;171:135-54.
12. Mellin G. Correlation of spinal mobility with degree of chronic low back pain after correction for age and anthropometric factors. Spine. 1987; 12(5):464-8.
13. Hu HY, Chou Y, et al. Association between obesity and injury among Tiawanese adults. Int J Obesity. 2009;33(8):878-84.
14. Ament PW, Bertolino JG, Liszewski JL. Clinically significant drug interactions. Am Fam Physician. 2000;61(6):1745-54.
15. Shorr RI, Ray WA, Daugherty JR, et al. Concomitant use of nonsteroidal anti-inflammatory drugs and oral anticoagulants places elderly persons at high risk for hemorrhagic peptic ulcer disease.Arch Intern Medicine. 1993;153:1665-70.
16. Yildrim K, Deniz O, Gureser G, et al. Gabapentin monotherapy in patients with chronic radiculopathy: the efficacy and impact on life quality. Journal of Back Musculoskeletal Rehabilitation. 2009;22(1):17-20.
17. Rogawski MA, Loscher W. The neurobiology of antiepileptic drugs for treatment on nonepileptic conditions. Nat MED. 2004;10(7):685-92.
18. Moore RA, Wiffen PJ, Derry S, McQuay HJ. Gabapentin for chronic neuropathic pain and fibromyalgia in adults. Cochrane Database Syst Rev. 2011;(3):7938-39.
19. Maitland GD. Vertebral Manipulation. 5th edition. London: Butterworths; 1986.
20. Rademeyer I. Manual therapy for lumbar spinal stenosis: a comprehensive physical therapy approach. Phys Med Rehabil Clin N Am. 2003; 14(1):103-10.
21. Fritz J, Erhard R, Vignovic M. A non-surgical approach for patients with lumbar spinal stenosis. Journal Physical Therapy. 1997;77(9):962-73.
22. De Rosa CP, Porterfield JA. A physical therapy model for treatment of low back pain. J Phys Therapy. 1992;72:261-72.
23. Manchikanti L, Staats PJ, Vijay S, et al. Evidence based practice guidelines for interventional techniques in management of chronic spinal pain. Pain Physician. 2003;6:3-81.
24. Goodman BS, Dosecian Lyle WF, Mallenpati S. Complications and pitfalls of lumbar interlaminar and transforaminal epidural steroid injections. Current Review Musculoskeletal Medicine. 2008;1(3-4):212-22.

25. Okell RW, Sprigge JS. Unintentional dural puncture: a survey of recognition and management. Anaesthesia. 1987;42:1110-3.
26. Liu S, Carpenter RL, Neal JM. Epidural anesthesia and analgesia: their role in post operative outcome. Anesthiology. 1995;82(6):1474-1506.
27. Turnbull DK, Shephard DB. Post dural puncture headache: pathogenesis, prevention and treatment. Br J Anaesth. 2003:91(5):718-29.
28. Ahmed G, Arjang K, Mangar D. Post dural headache. Int J Gen Med. 2012;5:45-51. Published online January 2012.
29. Vakharia SB, Thomas DS, Rosenbaum AE, et al. Magnetic resonance imaging of cerebrospinal fluid leak and tamponade effect of blood patch in post dural headache. Anesth Analg. 1997;84(3);585-90.
30. Frank JE Falco, Ongewu Obi C, Lee Irwin Sr F, et al. Peripheral joint, soft tissue and spinal injection techniques. In: Braddom RL. Physical Medicine and Rehabilitation. 3rd edition. Philadelphia PA: Elsevier; 2007.p.550.
31. Windsor RE, Storm S, Sugar R. Prevention and management of complications from common spinal injections. Pain Physician. 2003;6:473-83.
32. Harlocher TT, Wedel DJ, Benzon H, et al. Regional anesthesia in the anticoagulated patient, defining the risks. Reg Anesth Pain Med. 2003;28:172-97.
33. Stoll A, Sanchez M. Epidural hematoma after epidural block, implications for its use in pain management. Surg Neurol. 2002;57:235-40.
34. Lawton MT, Porter RW, Heisserman JE. Surgical management of spinal epidural hematoma: relationship between surgical timing and neurological outcome. J Neurosurgery. 1995;83:1-7.
35. Manchikanti L, Abdi S, Atluri S, Benyamin RM, Boswell MV, Buenaventura RM, Bryce DA, Burks PA, Caraway DL et al. An update of comprehensive evidence-based guidelines for interventional techniques in chronic spinal pain. Part II: guidance and recommendations. Pain Physician. 2013 Apr.
36. Gogarten W, Vandermeulen E, Van Aken H, Kozek S, Llau JV, Samama CM; European Scoeity of Anaesthesiology. Regional anaesthesia and antithrombotic agents: recommendations of the European Society of Anaesthesiology. Eur J Anaesthesiol. 2010 Dec;27(12):999-1015, 16(2 Suppl):S49-283.
37. Sullivan WJ, Willick SE, Chira-Adisai W. Incidence of intravascular uptake in lumbar spinal injection procedures. Spine. 2000;25:481-6.
38. Mulroy MF. Systemic toxicity and cardiotoxicity from local anesthics incidence and prevention measures. Reg Anesth Pain Med. 2002;27:556-61.
39. Yilmaz M, Wong CA. Technique of neuroaxial anesthesia. In: Wong CA (Ed). Spinal and Epidural Anesthesia. 1st edition. New York: McGraw Hill Medical Companies; 2007.pp.27-74.
40. Rho ME, Tang CT. Phys Med Rehabil Clin N Am. 2011 Feb;22(1):139-48. Epub 2010 Dec 3.The efficacy of lumbar epidural steroid injections: transforaminal, interlaminar, and caudal approaches.

5

Coccygodynia

Michael J Mehnert, Ferheen Shamim, Patrick M Foye

CHIEF COMPLAINT

The patient complains about "tailbone pain".

HISTORY OF PRESENT ILLNESS

The patient is a 24-year-old female with no significant past medical history, who presents to the office. She reports the onset of tailbone pain approximately 18 months ago after she slipped on ice and landed on her tailbone. Initially she noted some bruising and soreness over the area but was told that she "did not break anything" after X-rays in the emergency room. She had severe pain with sitting and walking initially, though this has improved significantly with time and use of anti-inflammatories. She has had a persistent aching sensation of pain that is 2 out of 10 and mainly occurs when sitting in her car. She recently switched occupations and is now sitting and driving more, with pain that has now escalated to 8–10 out of 10. She has tried using a "donut" style tailbone cushion without relief. She also has pain with changing position from sitting to standing, and with sitting on softer surfaces more than firm ones. Sex and bowel movements reproduce some of her pain as well, and as per the patient, the area is actually tender. She has no genitourinary complaints and no changes in stool or bright red blood per rectum. There are no constitutional symptoms and no reports of radicular pain, numbness, tingling or weakness in the lower limbs.

She continues on occasional usage of Tylenol or nonsteroidal antiinflammatory drugs (NSAIDs) for pain. She is interested in additional information about her condition and other treatment options. She has also considered seeing a pelvic therapist.

PAST MEDICAL/SURGICAL HISTORY

Appendectomy as a teenager

REVIEW OF SYSTEMS

As above. In addition the patient has no history of pregnancy or childbirth. She reports normal menstrual periods for 5 days with a regular 28-day cycle and normal flow. She does not describe painful menses and has no history of endometriosis or other pelvic pathology. No prior urinary tract infections are described. She reports no vaginal discharge or dysuria.

FAMILY HISTORY

None significant

SOCIAL HISTORY

She consumes 1–2 drinks over the course of a weekend but no daily alcohol use. She denies any tobacco or other drug use. She works as a pharmaceutical sales representative.

CURRENT MEDICATIONS

Tylenol Extra-Strength, rarely over-the-counter Advil.

ALLERGIES

No known drug allergies.

The pain diagram of the patient is shown in Figure 5.1.

PHYSICAL EXAMINATION

Height: 5'8", Weight: 124 lbs, Body mass index (BMI): 18.9, Pulse: 70/min Blood pressure (BP): 118/72 mm Hg Respirations: 10/min.

This is an alert, awake and cooperative female. Nutrition and hygiene are well-maintained. She is in no acute distress. She ambulates with a normal gait and station and can do heel-and-toe walking. Coordination is intact.

Thoracolumbar spine examination demonstrates normal overlying skin without erythema, edema, or surgical scar. Range of motion is full and the area is nontender above the waist, including the lumbar paraspinals, facet joints and the quadratus lumborum. The spinous processes are nontender.

On inspection of the sacrum and coccygeal area, there is again normal overlying skin without erythema or bruising. There is focal tenderness to palpation over the distal coccyx that reproduces her usual pain. Pelvis/genital

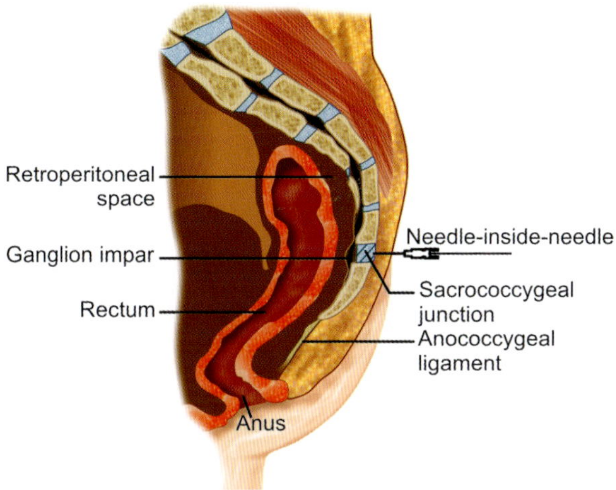

Fig. 5.1: Pain diagram of the patient

examination was not performed. There was no tenderness to palpation of the bilateral sacroiliac joints, piriformis muscles, or ischial bursae.

Neurological examination demonstrates 5/5 strength in the upper and lower limbs in all key myotomes tested. Sensory testing to light touch and pinprick is normal in the upper and lower limbs in all key dermatomes tested. Reflexes are 2+ and symmetric in the upper and lower limbs at the biceps, triceps, brachioradialis, patella and the Achilles.

Dural tension signs are negative in the lower limbs.

IMAGING

X-rays: Anterior-posterior (AP), lateral, flexion and extension views of the lumbar spine were normal. Disc height was well-maintained with normal lumbar lordosis. No instability is noted on flexion or extension.

Anterior-posterior and lateral views of the sacrum and coccyx were also obtained. There are three coccyx segments without evidence of fracture. Alignment is well-maintained.

DIAGNOSIS

Coccygodynia (coccyx pain) was diagnosed. The patient's symptoms are compatible with tailbone pain, or coccygodynia (also known as coccydynia). Though her X-rays are unremarkable, the patient has pain that occurs with prolonged sitting and with position changes, and she has focal tenderness to palpation over the coccyx.[1] She has symptoms that will occasionally occur with bowel movements or sexual activity. There is also a history of a preceding tailbone trauma, and though no discrete fracture has been identified, the patient did have a direct trauma that had reportedly caused temporary ecchymoses over this area. Post-traumatic instability or "luxation" of the coccygeal segments has been well-defined, and comparison of sitting and standing X-ray films may be useful in eliciting radiographic evidence of instability.[1-3]

DIFFERENTIAL DIAGNOSIS

The differential diagnosis would include other spinal causes of pain, such as perhaps a sacral fracture. Referred pain from the lumbar spine is less likely as the patient has no complaints of low back pain or radicular pain and there is a normal neurological examination. It may be prudent for this patient to be evaluated by her primary doctor or obstetrician/gynecologist (OBS/GYN) to rule-out intrapelvic pathology (ovarian cysts or perhaps endometriosis) but again, these diagnoses would be unlikely given that she is focally tender over the coccyx area and also when the history of her prior tailbone injury is taken into consideration. Possible malignancy should be considered, and if there is a reasonable suspicion an MRI should be obtained.[4,5]

COCCYGODYNIA

Coccyx pain has been well-documented.[1,6] The coccyx is named after a cuckoo, as it can be said to resemble a bird's beak in appearance.[7] It exists as the most inferiorly-located bony spinal segments, articulating with the sacrum (at the sacrococcygeal junction) and with each other (via the intercoccygeal junctions). Often, the segments of the coccyx are connected with a thin vestigial or fibrocartilage disc space. Range of motion of the coccyx exists in only one plane with flexion and extension (or, in some cases, no mobility)[2,3] occurring during the process of sitting as weight is distributed among the ischial tuberosities and the pelvic support structures.

Coccyx pain can occur from direct trauma or injury. Though a true bony fracture is a rare entity,[1] luxation or instability can result with or without a direct trauma or from repetitive microtrauma from sitting, abnormal mechanics with sitting, or anatomic variability in the coccyx itself.

Just anterior to the upper coccyx or the lower sacrum (within the retrorectal space)[8-10] lies the midline ganglion impar ("unpaired ganglion"). Also known as the ganglion of Walther, it is the most inferiorly-located ganglia of the sympathetic nervous system. Much like the stellate ganglion and the lumbar sympathetic ganglion, this structure is postulated to cause "sympathetic pain", though in the pelvic area. A mechanism of hyperactivity or hypersensitivity of the ganglion impar has been postulated as a cause for sympathetically maintained tailbone pain that will respond to treatment directed at the ganglion.[11] Blockade of the ganglion impar has been reportedly effective in controlling pelvic pain and coccygodynia.[8,9,12-14]

TREATMENT OPTIONS

The patient has already trialed a "donut" style coccyx cushion. A "wedge" type of cushion with a coccyx relief cutout could also be trialed. She has taken acetaminophen and nonsteroidal anti-inflammatory drugs (NSAIDs) with some relief, though this is incomplete.

Unfortunately, this patient has increased her driving as a result of a change in her occupation. She may benefit from trying to avoid sitting on softer surfaces if possible, as this seems to increase her pain as well.

Physical therapy options exist, both in the form of pelvic therapy with an experienced and skilled therapist, and also in the form of manual manipulation. These options could be discussed with the patient prior to pursuing interventional management.[15]

Coccygectomy has also been described as a treatment option, with some success in carefully selected patients. This generally should be considered a last resort only after other interventional treatments fail, and the literature supports better outcomes in patients who are severely debilitated by their pain.[16]

INTERVENTIONAL OPTIONS

From an interventional standpoint, a ganglion impar injection has been described as being useful for treatment of pelvic pain, particularly when it is thought to be sympathetically mediated. A reliable approach includes accessing the ganglion impar by inserting a needle through the vestigial disc space (intercoccygeal or sacrococcygeal) (Fig. 5.2) and applying local anesthetic to the ganglion.[8,12]

Various injection techniques have been described, including an initial "blind" injection. Modern techniques via a variety of approaches employ fluoroscopic guidance with usage of contrast media for accurate medication placement and to minimize the risk of adverse reactions.[9,10,17-20] Much like a cervical or lumbar sympathetic ganglion blockade, the structure is anesthetized with short- and/or long-acting anesthetic. The patient should report immediate relief of pain with provocative activity (generally sitting) after the injection.

A published case series of ganglion impar blocks for patients diagnosed with persistent coccygodynia demonstrated that all injections provided some level of relief in these patients, with results varying from 20% to 75% pain relief and most patients responding with 50–75% relief. Repeat injections were often helpful for patients with incomplete relief.[13] A patient with complete, lasting relief after one block has also been reported.[14]

Radiofrequency neurotomy of the ganglion impar has also been explored,[21,22] and may be an option for recalcitrant pain that responds temporarily to

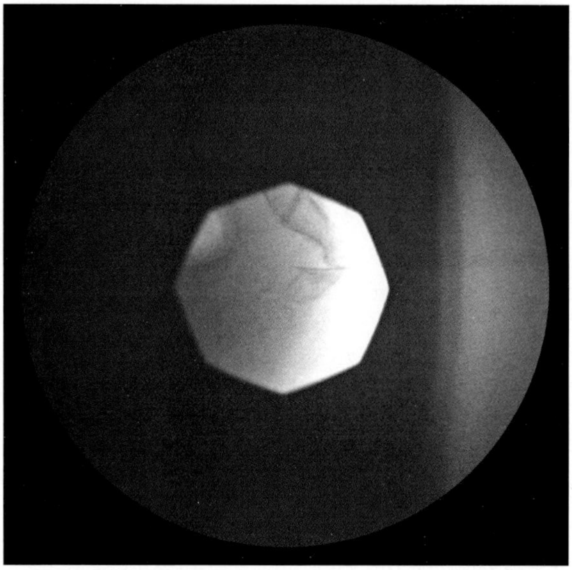

Fig. 5.2: Lateral view of the needle traversing the inter-coccygeal junction and placed just beyond the anterior margin of the coccyx, prior to contrast injection

sympathetic blocks. The procedure is challenging both due to the proximity of the ganglion to delicate visceral structures such as the rectum, bowel, and anus, and also due to the difficulty of placing a probe at the target site. Chemodenervation with phenol or neurotoxic agents has also been established but is not in wide use.[6]

Some practitioners have also advocated for the use of caudal epidural steroid injections for tailbone pain, though little published data exist to support their use.[23]

PLAN

The above treatment options were discussed in detail with the patient. She expressed a lack of interest in surgery and frustration with her increasing pain and resulting functional deficits, particularly with regard to her recent job change and the need to drive longer distances. A plan was made to move forward with a fluoroscopically-guided ganglion impar block (sympathetic nerve block) for better pain control and sitting tolerance.

PROCEDURE

Coccyx injection/ganglion impar sympathetic block with fluoroscopic guidance.

Indications

Please refer to prior office notes for details. The patient is being treated for a diagnosis of coccygodynia (tailbone pain). The patient has failed to respond to oral anti-inflammatory medications and use of pressure-relief cushions to relieve pain over the coccyx area. A decision was made to proceed with a fluoroscopically-guided ganglion impar injection for diagnostic and possibly therapeutic purposes.

The patient was informed of the risks and benefits of the procedure, as well as alternative treatments. All questions were answered prior to proceeding. The patient expressed understanding and gave informed written consent.

Preoperative Diagnosis

Coccygodynia (tailbone pain)

Postoperative Diagnosis

Same as preoperative diagnosis

Procedure Performed

- Sympathetic nerve block at the anterior coccyx (ganglion impar block)
- Fluoroscopic guidance/localization.

The patient was taken into the fluoroscopy suite and was placed prone on the examination table. The overlying skin was prepped and draped in the usual sterile fashion. Under AP and intermittent fluoroscopic guidance, the sacrococcygeal junction was identified, and a lateral view was used to begin the procedure. The overlying skin was marked using a metal pointer for radiographic guidance. Local anesthetic (1% lidocaine without preservative buffered) was administered to anesthetize the skin and subcutaneous tissues.

Next, a 25-gauge, 3½-inch sterile spinal needle was inserted via the (sacrococcygeal, 1st intracoccygeal, etc.) junction using intermittent fluoroscopic guidance under AP and lateral views. The needle was then placed appropriately just at the anterior aspect of the coccyx and this was confirmed by lateral fluoroscopy. Next, aspiration revealed no return of blood or other fluid. Then, a solution of 2 mL of water-soluble nonionic contrast media was then injected via the spinal needle. Fluoroscopy on the lateral view once again confirmed that the needle tip was located at the anterior aspect of the coccyx/coccygeal junction and there was longitudinal spread of the contrast just anterior to the sacrum and coccyx, thus covering the ganglion impar. There was no evidence of contrast filling in the rectum. Under live fluoroscopy, no evidence of vascular uptake was noted. Proper placement was also confirmed in the AP view. Next, a solution of 4 mL of

1% lidocaine without preservative and 6 mL of 0.25% bupivacaine without preservative was injected via the spinal needle. Fluoroscopy showed contrast washout, further confirming good placement of the injected solution. The needle was withdrawn and good hemostasis was noted.

Immediately upon sitting up from the procedure, the patient reported ____% relief. The patient understands that when the nerve blocks wear off, the coccygodynia may return, but usually it is less severe than prior to the injections. If additional relief is still needed, the blocks can be repeated for additional benefit.

The patient tolerated the procedure well and without complications.

The patient was instructed to apply ice over the injection site for 10–15 minutes for the next 24–48 hours. A postprocedure instruction sheet was given.

Ganglion impar injection images are shown in Figures 5.3 to 5.8.

CONCERNS, PITFALLS AND TIPS

- Care should be taken to advance the needle gently and slowly through the sacrococcygeal junction or intercoccygeal space. Remember that the rectum and visceral bowel structures are in close proximity to and just anterior to the bony structures; avoiding perforation should obviously be a paramount concern.
- The lateral coccyx view is ideal to begin the procedure, however, may sometimes be a difficult fluoroscopy view to optimize. The bony sacrum

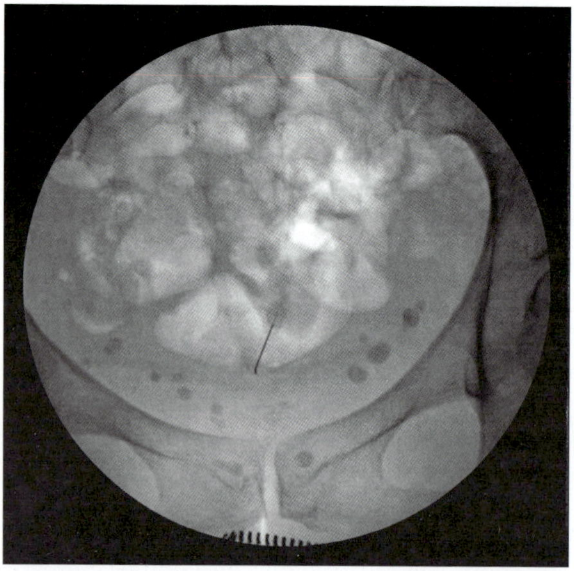

Fig. 5.3: A-P view of needle in place for a ganglion impar injection. Note the difficulty identifying detailed bony anatomy given the viceral structures and bowel gas

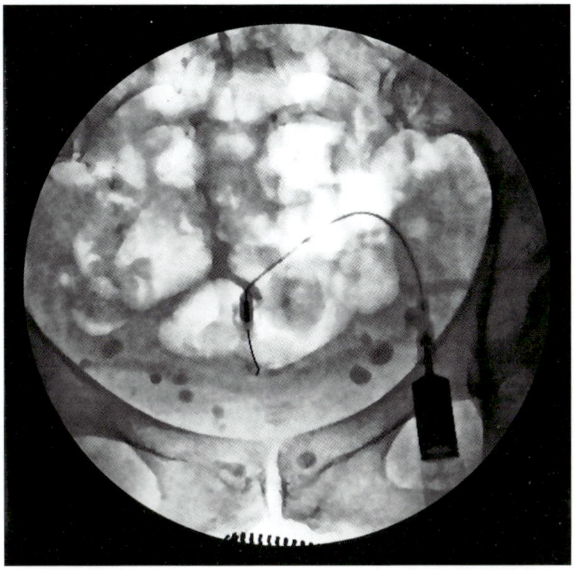

Fig. 5.4: A-P view of the needle in place after contrast injection

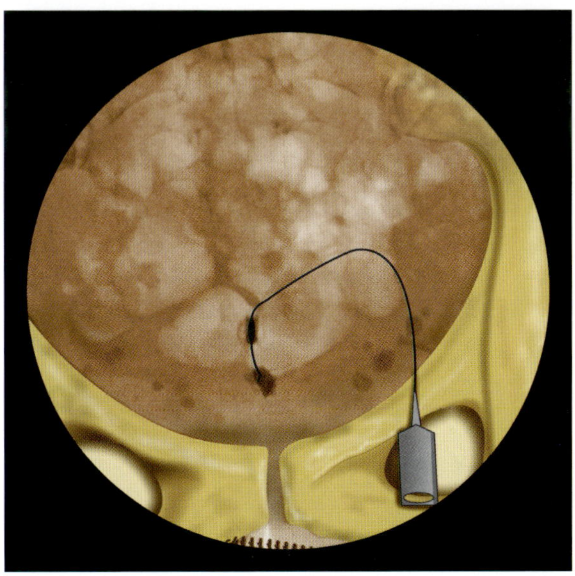

Fig. 5.5: A-P view of the needle in place after contrast injection (rendering to show bony anatomy)

and coccyx exist as a thin plane between a top layer of skin and overlying air and the bottom layer of gaseous visceral structures such as the rectum and bowel. In addition, the larger nearby bony structures in the pelvis and the spine may limit visibility of the relatively small coccyx segments. Also, the majority of the field will often contain air above and below the bony

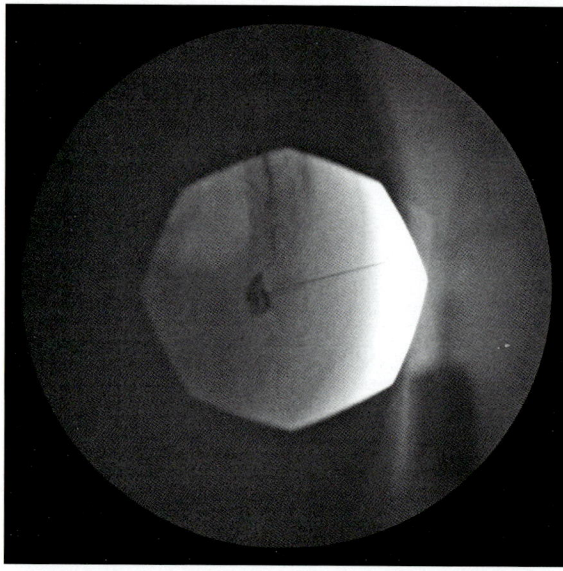

Fig. 5.6: Initial contrast injection showing appropriate spread of injectate in the retroperitoneal space

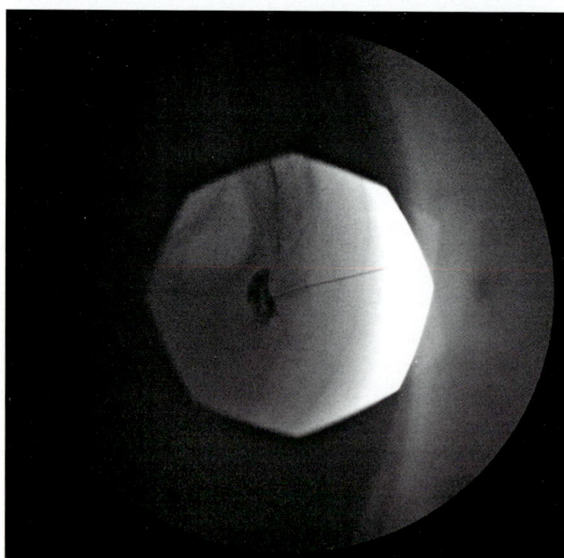

Fig. 5.7: Additional injection of contrast showing injectate spreading along the anterior aspect of the coccyx in the retroperitoneal space, thus covering the ganglion impar

structures and may result in "washing out" of the image. As a result, extra care should be taken to optimize the lateral view with "coning down" the field and localizing/marking the injection site with a metal pointer prior to beginning the procedure.

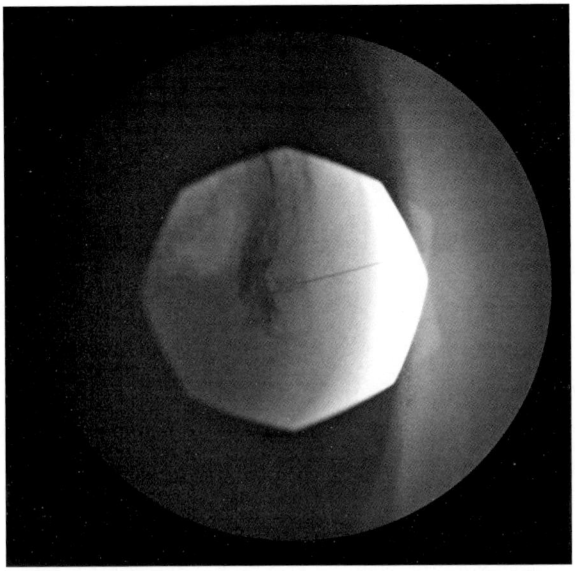

Fig. 5.8: "Washout" image of the contrast being diluted as madication is injected and further covers the target location

- Sterile gauze may be placed at the top of the patient's gluteal fold to help distract the soft tissue and better visualize the injection site and also to prevent betadine or other antiseptic solution from flowing beyond the target sterile area.
- In addition, it is often beneficial to direct the needle for the local anesthetic right down to the posterior aspect of the bony sacrum/coccyx superior to the target injection junction to administer local anesthetic over the traversing posterior fibers of the somatic coccygeal nerve. This may make the remainder of the procedure less painful for the patient.
- It is recommended that the operator attempts to access the ganglion impar by traversing the vestigial disc space with a small gauge needle, optimally a 25-gauge, 3.5-inch or 2.0-inch needle. If the target junction is significantly degenerative or sclerotic, a larger gauge needle could be attempted prior to attempting access at a different level. Alternatively, gentle pressure downward on the distal coccyx may also theoretically help to distract the posterior entry to the sacrococcygeal or intracoccygeal junction. Foye et al. have also described an alternate "corkscrew" paracoccygeal injection approach[10] if the fibrocartilage junction cannot be penetrated.
- At times, if the target sacrococcygeal or intracoccygeal junction appears to be significantly degenerative or arthritic, one could also inject corticosteroid into the vestigial disc space/junctional space (Fig. 5.9). Efficacy of this intervention has not been well established.

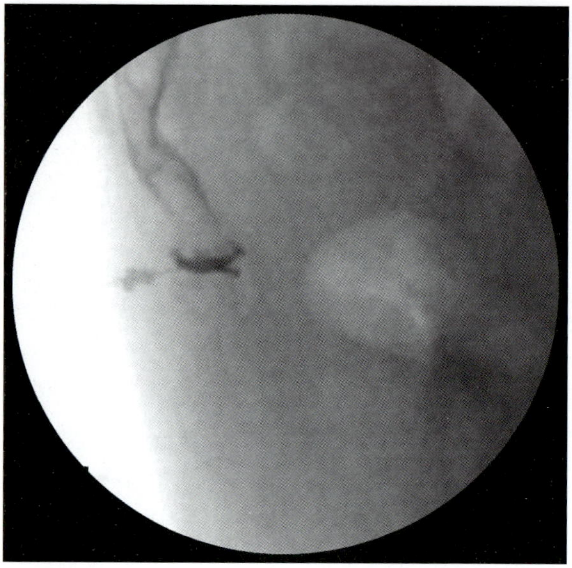

Fig. 5.9: Coccygeal discography

REFERENCES

1. Maigne JY. Coccydynia. In: Slipman CW, Derby R, Simeone FA, Mayer TG (Eds). Interventional Spine: An Algorithmic Approach. Philadelphia, PA: Saunders Elsevier; 2008. pp.1289-97.
2. Maigne JY, Molinie V, Fautrel B. Anatomie des disques sacro et inter-coccygiens. Revue de Medecine Orthopedique. 1992;28:34-5.
3. Maigne JY, Lagauche D, Doursounian L. Instability of the coccyx in coccydynia. J Bone Joint Surg. 2000;82B:1038-41.
4. Maigne JY, Pigeau I, Roger B. Magnetic resonance imaging findings in the painful adult coccyx. Eur Spine J. Published online February 2012.
5. Foye PM. Coccyx pain diagnostic workup: necessity of MRI in detecting malignancy present with tailbone pain. Am J Phys Med Rehabil. 2002; 89:S33.
6. Howorth B. The painful coccyx. Clin Orthop. 1959;14:145-50.
7. Sugar O. Coccyx, the bone named for a bird. Spine. 1995;20:379-83.
8. Plancarte R, Amescua C, Patt RB, et al. Presacral blockade of the ganglion of Walther (ganglion impar). Anesthesiology. 1990;73(3A):A751.
9. Toshniwal GR, Dureja GP, Prashanth SM. Trans-sacrococcygeal approach to ganglion impar block for management of chronic perineal pain: a prospective observational study. Pain Physician. 2007;10:661-6.
10. Foye PM, Patel SL. Paracoccygeal corkscrew approach to ganglion impar injections for tailbone pain. Pain Pract. 2009;9(4):317-21.
11. Oh CS, Chung IH, Ji HJ, et al. Clinical implications of topographic anatomy on the ganglion impar. Anesthesiology. 2004;101(1):249-50.
12. Foye PM, Kirschner JS, Furman MB. Ganglion impar injection. In: Furman MB, Lee TS, Berkwits L (Eds). Atlas of Image-Guided Spinal Procedures. Philadelphia, PA: Elsevier Saunders; 2013. pp. 63-71.

13. Buttaci CJ, Foye PM, Stitik TP. Coccydynia successfully treated with ganglion impar blocks: a case series. Am J Phys Med Rehabil. 2005;84(3):218.
14. Foye PM, Buttaci CJ, Stitik TP, et al. Successful injection for coccyx pain. Am J Phys Med Rehabil. 2006;85:783-4.
15. Maigne JY, Chatellier G. Comparison of three manual coccydynia treatments: a pilot study. Spine. 2001;26:479-84.
16. Balain B, Eisenstein SM, Alo GO, et al. Coccygectomy for coccydynia: case series and review of literature. Spine. 2006;31(13):E414-E420.
17. Foye PM. Ganglion impar blocks via coccygeal versus sacrococcygeal joints. Reg Anesth Pain Med. 2008;33(3):279-80.
18. Foye PM. New approaches to ganglion impar blocks via coccygeal joints. Reg Anesth Pain Med. 2007;32(3):269.
19. Kuthuru M, Kabbara AI, Oldenburg P, et al. Coccygeal pain relief after trans-sacrococcygeal block of the ganglion impar under fluoroscopy: a case report. Arch Phys Med Rehabil. 2003;84(9):E24.
20. Kabbara AI. Trans-sacrococcygeal ganglion impar block for postherpetic neuralgia. Anesthesiology. 2005;103(1):211-2.
21. Atim A, Ergin A, Bilgiç S, et al. Pulsed radio-frequency in the treatment of coccygodynia. Agri. 2011;23(1):1-6.
22. Reig E, Abejón D, Del Pozo C, et al. Thermocoagulation of the ganglion impar or ganglion of Walther: description of a modified approach. Preliminary results in chronic, nononcological pain. Pain Pract. 2005;5(2):103-10.
23. Foye PM, Buttaci CJ, Sorensen MK, et al. Coccyx Pain—eMedicine Online Publication. Accessed online 2013 at http://emedicine.medscape.com/article/309486-overview.

6

Lumbar Facet Syndrome

Jeremy Simon, Kelly Williams

CHIEF COMPLAINT

The patient complains about lower back pain.

HISTORY OF PRESENT ILLNESS

A 61-year-old right-handed male presents with a 10 year history of mild intermittent lower back pain, progressively worsening over the last 3 years without an inciting event. It is predominantly midline and slightly to the lower right side of his back with occasional radiation to the buttock and right thigh, never below the knee. Extension, prolonged standing, twisting and lifting aggravate the pain. It is worse in the morning with associated stiffness in the lower back, but has become a constant deep, dull ache throughout the day and a "tight feeling in the muscles" in the lower back. The pain is reduced with sitting and forward flexion. It can be sharp when extending, twisting and lifting. There is no associated unintentional weight loss or weight gain, fevers, chills or night sweats, weakness, numbness, tingling, or night pain. There is no radiating pain down either leg. He is employed as a plumber and has worked for 40 years.

Treatments to date include nonsteroidal anti-inflammatory medications and muscle relaxers with mild relief, physical therapy with a flexion bias and core strengthening with mild relief, transcutaneous electrical nerve stimulation (TENS), heating pads, chiropractic, acupuncture, trigger point injections, and massage therapy with modest relief. He is coming to your office for a more complete understanding of his problem and to explore the possibility of interventional treatments for his pain.

PAST MEDICAL HISTORY

Hypertension, hyperlipidemia

PAST SURGICAL HISTORY

None

REVIEW OF SYSTEMS

Otherwise negative

FAMILY HISTORY

Parents alive with no medical issues.

SOCIAL HISTORY

Drinks 1–2 glasses of beer at night, smokes one pack of cigarettes/day, denies illicit drugs. Employed as a plumber, full time, no workmen's compensation claims.

CURRENT MEDICATIONS

Ibuprofen 200 mg bid prn, cyclobenzaprine 10 mg qhs prn, lisinopril 10 mg qDay.

ALLERGIES

None

The pain diagram of the patient is shown in Figure 6.1.

PHYSICAL EXAMINATION

Height: 5'10", Weight: 270 lbs, Pulse: 82/min, BP: 145/85 mm Hg, Respirations: 16/min.

General: Pleasant, cooperative, looks stated age, obese, in no distress.

Gait and tandem gait stable, with *slight forward flexion*. Romberg sign is negative. Able to heel walk and toe walk without difficulty. Pulses are 2+ in the radial and dorsalis pedis arteries. Babinski testing reveals downgoing toes bilaterally. Slump test and supine straight leg raise to 90° are negative bilaterally. Negative femoral nerve stretch test bilaterally. No palpable step-off in the lumbar spine. No tenderness over the lumbar spinous processes. No palpable scoliotic curve. *There is palpable muscle spasm in the lumbar*

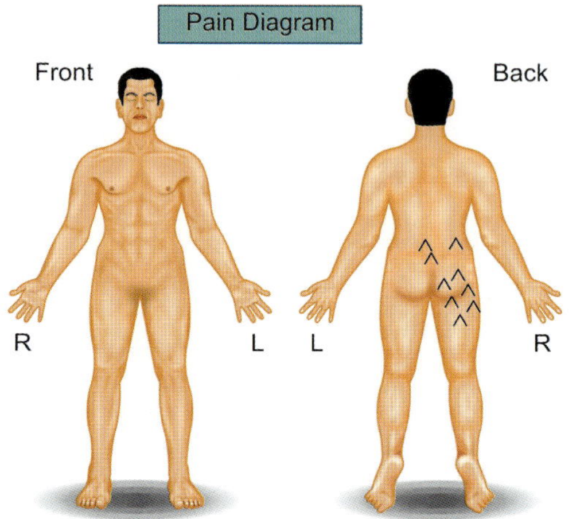

Using the symbols below, the location and type of pain sensations are marked on the diagrams. All the affected areas are included.

TYPE OF SENSATIONS

Aching	^ ^ ^ ^ ^ ^
Sharp or stabbing	X X X X X X
Burning	//////////
Pins and needles	---------------
Numbness	0 0 0 0 0 0

Fig. 6.1: Pain diagram of the patient

paraspinals and tenderness. Patrick's test is negative bilaterally, but provokes some mild reproduction of pain in the lower back on the right. Internal rotation of the hips does not cause pain. No tenderness to palpation over the bilateral trochanteric bursae. Negative Gaenslen's sign, negative Thomas test, negative Ober's test bilaterally. No tenderness over the sacroiliac joints. Manual muscle testing in the lower limbs reveals 5/5 bilateral hip flexors, quadriceps, tibialis anterior, extensor hallucis longus, and gastrocsoleus. Sensory examination to light touch and pinprick is normal in the lower extremity dermatomes. Proprioception is intact at the great toes bilaterally. Normal muscle tone. Reflexes are 2+ in patellae, medial hamstrings and Achilles tendons. No ankle clonus bilaterally. *Lumbar range of motion is reduced in extension and the end limits of flexion. There is reproduction of typical pain with extension and extension/rotation to the right. Posterior-anterior pressure over the L4-L5 and L5-S1 segments on the right cause reproduction of pain.*

IMAGING

Lumbar spine X-rays: Anterior-posterior, lateral, flexion and extension lumbar X-rays reveal moderate disc space narrowing at L4-L5 and L5-S1. Normal segmentation, no spondylolisthesis or scoliosis.

Magnetic resonance imaging: Disc degeneration at L4-L5, L5-S1. Broad-based disc bulge at L5-S1 without neural compression. Prominent facet arthropathy, right greater than left, at L4-L5 and L5-S1.

DIAGNOSIS

Lumbar zygapophysial joint (facet) syndrome—likely involving the right L4-L5 and L5-S1 zygapophysial joints.

TREATMENT OPTIONS

Lifestyle modifications should be emphasized. Obesity adds load to the spine and may contribute to his pain. Poor conditioning and lack of adequate core strength can also play a role.[1,2] Smoking cessation and healthy lifestyle should be promoted.[3-5]

Proper ergonomics and lifting mechanics should be emphasized. Potential referral for "back school" is indicated due to the physicality of his work.[6] Job satisfaction and the amount of strain on his lower back may impact his outcome and the potential for reoccurrence.[7]

One might consider increasing the ibuprofen dose to 600–800 mg to achieve the anti-inflammatory affects not seen at 200 mg, as well as increasing the frequency to three times a day. Prior to suggesting this, a clearance from the patient's primary care physician would be advisable due to the elevated blood pressure. This may be a spurious reading, but if he has hypertension, increasing the nonsteroidal anti-inflammatory drugs (NSAIDs) may contribute to higher blood pressures.[8]

Conflicting data exists regarding the role of spinal manipulation in the setting of lumbar facet syndrome.[9,10] Possible mechanisms of pain relief include restoration of normal motion through physiological barriers, the gait theory of pain, endorphin release, and stimulation of joint mechanoreceptors that reflexively alters alpha motor neuron excitability.[11] Neurophysiologic studies of facet joint strain during manipulation suggest its safety.[12] Some studies see a greater benefit in particular subgroups like facet syndrome as opposed to spinal stenosis or radiculopathy.[11] Potential techniques include myofascial release, soft tissue, strain-counterstrain, muscle energy, and high-velocity low amplitude maneuvers.[13] Overall, in experienced hands, manipulation is an accepted and safe treatment option in the setting of benign low back pain and may be considered in this case.

His symptoms are consistent with lumbar zygapophysial joint syndrome. Pain associated with extension and extension-rotation are typical findings. Physical examination is neither sensitive nor specific for this entity.[14] Midline lower back pain with a lack of a radicular component also makes this diagnosis more likely. It is not unusual for pain to radiate into the posterior thigh or the flank.[14] Pain maps have been described corresponding

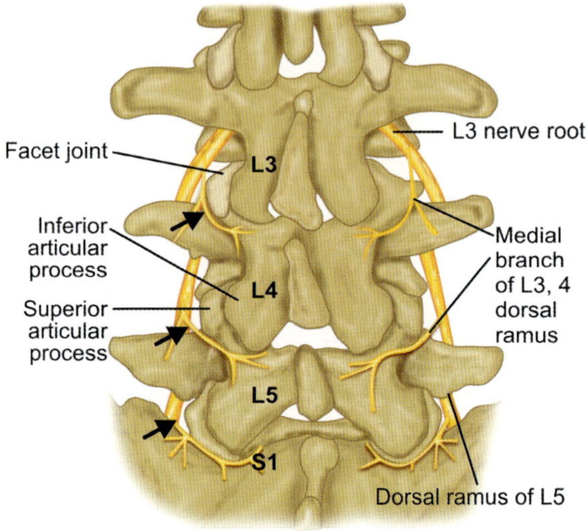

Fig. 6.2: Medial branch anatomy of the lumbar zygapophysial joint

to different joints involved.[15,16] Sacroiliac joint dysfunction is less likely. This is due to the primary location in the midline and not the buttocks as well as the lack of a groin component. Discogenic low back pain is also unlikely as the pain is relieved with sitting and aggravated with extension; the reverse is usually the case with internal disc disruption syndrome.[17]

The nerve supply to the lumbar zygapophysial joint is well described.[18,19] Two medial branch nerves emanating from the dorsal ramus supply each joint. The nomenclature can be confusing as the superior aspect of the joint is supplied by the nerve from above and the inferior by that below (Fig. 6.2). For example, the L4-L5 zygapophysial joint is supplied by the L3 and L4 medial branch nerves. The L5-S1 zygapophysial joint is supplied by the L4 medial branch nerve and the L5 dorsal ramus.

INTERVENTIONAL OPTIONS

The lumbar zygapophysial joints may be addressed by injection via an intra-articular approach or by "blocking" (anesthetizing) the nerves that supply them (Figs 6.3 to 6.5). Long-term benefit has not been proven with intra-injections of steroid and anesthetic.[20,21] Consideration to an intra-articular injection may be given, as medial branch blockade in theory does not offer therapeutic affects. In cases with severe osteoarthritis, an intra-articular injection may not be possible and medial branch block may be the only option. Some authors have noted up to 3 months of relief with medial branch blocks, but the primary indication for blocks is diagnostic.[22]

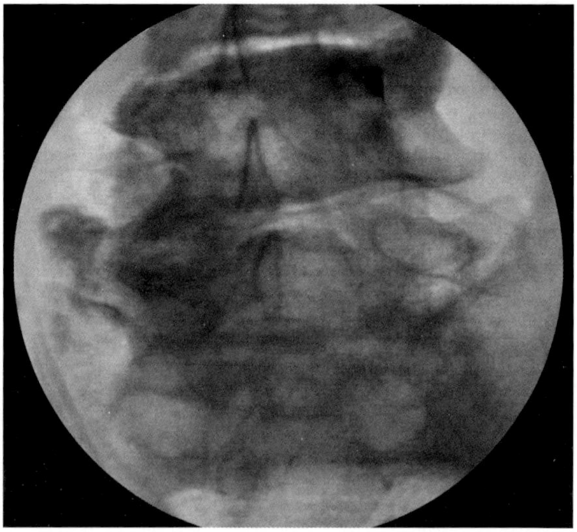

Fig. 6.3: L3 medial branch block

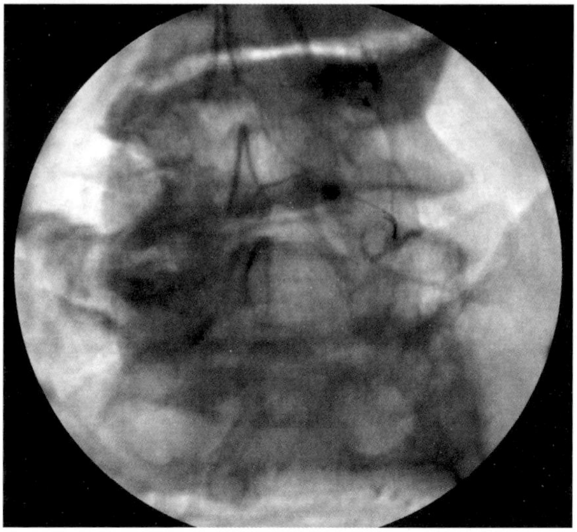

Fig. 6.4: L4 medial branch block

The International Spine Intervention Society (ISIS) recommends a two positive block paradigm for confirmation of the diagnosis.[23,24] Some practitioners may include one intra-articular injection and one medial branch block; two medial branch blocks are considered the standard. The injections are performed in conjunction with a pain diary. The patient's typical pain should be reduced between 50% and 100% depending on the criteria the physician uses to be considered positive.[23,25] The relief should correspond to the duration of the anesthetic used if the effects are temporary. There should

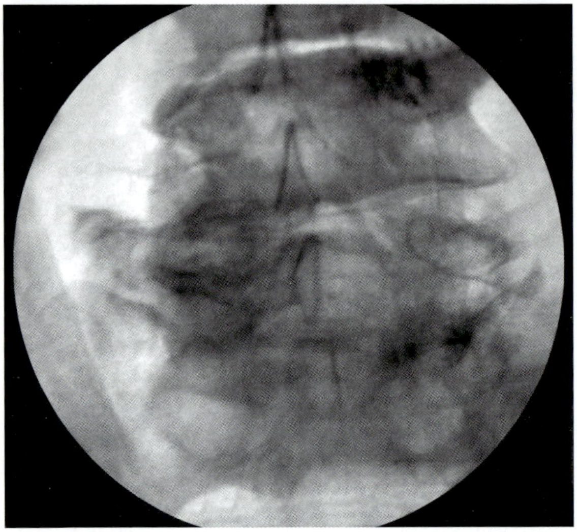

Fig. 6.5: L5 dorsal ramus block

be significantly less pain or no pain with typical aggravating activities while the anesthetic is on board and documentation should be made of these activities in the pain diary.

Lumbar medial branch radiofrequency ablation is a method for potentially giving longer-term relief of zygapophysial joint mediated pain. Relief is typically 12 months or more.[26,27] The procedure is performed in the outpatient setting with the use of special insulated radiofrequency needles with exposed active tips placed under fluoroscopic guidance over the regions where the medial branch nerves reside. The inner cannula (stylet) is replaced with a heating electrode that makes contact with the active tip. A grounding pad is placed on the patient and the probes are connected to a radiofrequency generator. This device also monitors impedance and temperature. It allows the delivery of radiofrequency energy directly to the needle tips.

Once the needles are in the correct position, the medial branch nerves should be stimulated one by one to assure that no radicular spread is obtained. This is performed by first using a sensory stimulation at 50 Hz, which may cause reproduction of typical low back pain in the absence of radicular spread. It is then followed by a motor stimulation at 2 Hz, which should cause contraction of the multifidii in the absence of contraction of lower limb muscles.

Once all impedances, pictures and stimulations are ideal, a lesioning protocol is then performed. The ideal temperature should be at 80°C for 90 seconds. Many authors advocate rotating the needles after the first cycle and repeating the lesioning 1–2 more times for an additional 60–90 seconds to assure maximal damage to the nerve. Up to four medial branch nerves may be lesioned at once with many of the newer machines.

SAMPLE PROCEDURE NOTES

Lumbar Intra-articular Zygapophysial Joint Injection

Informed consent for the procedure was obtained. The risks, benefits and alternative options were discussed. The risks include, but are not limited to, death, paralysis, allergic reaction, syncope, arrhythmia, cardiac or respiratory arrest, spinal cord injury, worse pain, scar formation, bleeding, epidural hematoma and infection. The patient was prepped and draped in a sterile fashion while in the prone position. All vital signs and oxygen saturation were monitored prior to, during and after the procedure.

The C-arm was positioned so that the region overlying the right L4-L5 and L5-S1 zygapophysial joints were visualized. The soft tissues overlying these structures were infiltrated with 4–6 cc of 1% lidocaine without epinephrine. A 25-gauge spinal needle was inserted into the superior aspect of each of the above mentioned zygapophysial joints. After negative aspirate for blood or cerebrospinal fluid (CSF), a small amount of nonionic contrast was injected and flow of contrast was noted. Radiographs were obtained for documentation purposes. The injectate consisting of steroid and lidocaine was administered into both joints.

The patient tolerated the procedure well and was discharged after an appropriate period of observation. If there are any complications, the patient was instructed by the authors to call them. The patient is to follow up with the physician as noted above within 2–3 weeks.

Lumbar Medial Branch Block (Zygapophysial Joint Nerve Block)

The C-arm was positioned so that the L5 vertebrae and sacral ala were identified. The soft tissues overlying these structures were anesthetized with 4–6 cc of 1% lidocaine without epinephrine.

At the L5 vertebrae, a 25-gauge spinal needle was advanced down under oblique view to the junction of the superior articular process and transverse process of the vertebra. This corresponds to the L4 medial branch nerve.

At the sacral ala, a 25-gauge spinal needle was advanced down to the junction of the sacral ala and the superior articular process of S1. This corresponds to the dorsal ramus of L5.

An anterior-posterior (AP) projection was used to confirm the positions. After negative aspirate for blood or CSF, a small amount of nonionic contrast was injected and flow of contrast was noted at each level, care given to assess for vascular flow. Radiographs were obtained for documentation purposes. The anesthetic was administered at both levels.

The patient tolerated the procedure well and was discharged after an appropriate period of observation. If there are any complications, the patient was instructed by the authors to call them. The patient is to follow up with the physician as noted above within 1–2 weeks.

The patient was also given a pain diary and was instructed to note the pain level and activities at the time of entering the data for the day of the procedure. The patient will have to bring this data to the follow-up appointment for diagnostic purposes.

Informed consent for the procedure was obtained. The risks, benefits and alternative options were discussed. The risks include, but are not limited to, death, paralysis, allergic reaction, syncope, arrhythmia, cardiac or respiratory arrest, spinal cord injury, worse pain, scar formation, bleeding, epidural hematoma and infection. The patient was prepped and draped in a sterile fashion while in the prone position. A grounding pad was placed on the patient. All vital signs were monitored prior to, during and after the procedure. Oxygen saturation was also monitored and noted to be greater than or equal to 94% throughout the procedure. Cardiac monitoring revealed normal sinus rhythm.

The C-arm was positioned so that the appropriate vertebral levels for the above mentioned zygapophysial joint nerves were visualized. The soft tissues overlying these structures were infiltrated with 4–6 cc of 1% lidocaine without epinephrine.

For L4 medial branch nerve, the radiofrequency needle was advanced down to the junction of the superior articular process and the transverse process via an oblique approach.

For the L5 dorsal ramus, the radiofrequency spinal needle was advanced down to the junction of the sacral ala and the superior articular process of S1.

Lateral and AP views were obtained to confirm safe and accurate placement. Then at each level, the radiofrequency needle stylet was replaced by the radiofrequency heating electrode. Sensory and motor test stimulation at 50 Hz and 2 Hz respectively was performed at both levels to ensure no radicular sensations and to obtain maximal multifidii contractions. After confirmation, 1 cc of 1% lidocaine without epinephrine was injected at both levels. Subsequently at each level, lesioning was done for approximately 90 seconds at 80°C. The lesioning was repeated two times at each level for approximately 90 seconds. Radiographs were obtained for documentation purposes.

The patient tolerated the procedure well and was discharged after an appropriate period of observation. If there are any complications, the patient was instructed by the authors to call them. The patient is to follow up with the physician as noted above within 2–3 weeks.

REFERENCES

1. Willemink MJ, van Es HW, Helmhout PH, et al. The effects of dynamic isolated lumbar extensor training on lumbar multifidus functional cross-sectional area and functional status of patients with chronic nonspecific low back pain. Spine. 2012;37:E1651-8.
2. Heuch I, Hagen K, Heuch I, et al. The impact of body mass index on the prevalence of low back pain: the HUNT study. Spine. 2010;35:764-8.
3. Behrend C, Prasarn M, Coyne E, et al. Smoking cessation related to improved patient-reported pain scores following spinal care. The Journal of Bone and Joint Surgery, American volume; 2012.
4. van Oostrom SH, Monique Verschuren WM, de Vet HC, et al. Ten year course of low back pain in an adult population-based cohort—the Doetinchem cohort study. European Journal of Pain. 2011;15:993-8.
5. Bjorck-van Dijken C, Fjellman-Wiklund A, Hildingsson C. Low back pain, lifestyle factors and physical activity: a population based-study. Journal of Rehabilitation Medicine: Official Journal of the UEMS European Board of Physical and Rehabilitation Medicine. 2008;40:864-9.
6. Sahin N, Albayrak I, Durmus B, et al. Effectiveness of back school for treatment of pain and functional disability in patients with chronic low back pain: a randomized controlled trial. Journal of Rehabilitation Medicine : Official Journal of the UEMS European Board of Physical and Rehabilitation Medicine. 2011;43:224-9.
7. Courvoisier DS, Genevay S, Cedraschi C, et al. Job strain, work characteristics and back pain: a study in a university hospital. European Journal of Pain. 2011;15:634-40.
8. Aljadhey H, Tu W, Hansen RA, et al. Comparative effects of non-steroidal anti-inflammatory drugs (NSAIDs) on blood pressure in patients with hypertension. BMC cardiovascular disorders. 2012;12:93.
9. Haigh R, Clarke AK. Effectiveness of rehabilitation for spinal pain. Clinical Rehabilitation. 1999;13 (Suppl 1):63-81.
10. Hadler NM, Curtis P, Gillings DB, et al. A benefit of spinal manipulation as adjunctive therapy for acute low-back pain: a stratified controlled trial. Spine. 1987;12:702-6.
11. Kirkaldy-Willis WH, Cassidy JD. Spinal manipulation in the treatment of low-back pain. Canadian family physician Medecin de famille canadien. 1985;31:535-40.
12. Ianuzzi A, Khalsa PS. Comparison of human lumbar facet joint capsule strains during simulated high-velocity, low-amplitude spinal manipulation versus physiological motions. The Spine Journal: Official Journal of the North American Spine Society. 2005;5:277-90.
13. Cyriax J. Manipulation trials. British Medical Journal. 1980;280:111.
14. van Kleef M, Vanelderen P, Cohen SP, et al. Pain originating from the lumbar facet joints. Pain Practice: the Official Journal of World Institute of Pain. 2010;10: 459-69.
15. Marks R. Distribution of pain provoked from lumbar facet joints and related structures during diagnostic spinal infiltration. Pain. 1989;39:37-40.
16. Windsor RE, King FJ, Roman SJ, et al. Electrical stimulation-induced lumbar medial branch referral patterns. Pain Physician. 2002;5:347-53.
17. Rengachary SS, Balabhadra RS. Black disc disease: a commentary. Neurosurgical Focus. 2002; 13:E14.

18. Bogduk N, Wilson AS, Tynan W. The human lumbar dorsal rami. Journal of Anatomy. 1982; 134:383-97.
19. Bogduk N. The innervation of the lumbar spine. Spine. 1983;8:286-93.
20. Falco FJ, Manchikanti L, Datta S, et al. An update of the effectiveness of therapeutic lumbar facet joint interventions. Pain Physician. 2012;15:E909-53.
21. Datta S, Lee M, Falco FJ, et al. Systematic assessment of diagnostic accuracy and therapeutic utility of lumbar facet joint interventions. Pain Physician. 2009;12:437-60.
22. Manchikanti L, Singh V, Falco FJ, et al. Lumbar facet joint nerve blocks in managing chronic facet joint pain: one-year follow-up of a randomized, double-blind controlled trial: Clinical Trial NCT00355914. Pain Physician. 2008; 11:121-32.
23. Derby R, Melnik I, Lee JE, et al. Correlation of lumbar medial branch neurotomy results with diagnostic medial branch block cutoff values to optimize therapeutic outcome. Pain Medicine. 2012;13:1533-46.
24. Bogduk N. Spinal Diagnostic and Treatment Procedures: Practice Guidelines, 1st edition. San Francisco, CA: International Spine Intervention Society; 2004.
25. Klessinger S. Zygapophysial joint pain in post lumbar surgery syndrome. The efficacy of medial branch blocks and radiofrequency neurotomy. Pain Medicine; 2012.
26. Speldewinde GC. Outcomes of percutaneous zygapophysial and sacroiliac joint neurotomy in a community setting. Pain Medicine. 2011;12:209-18.
27. Dreyfuss P, Halbrook B, Pauza K, et al. Efficacy and validity of radiofrequency neurotomy for chronic lumbar zygapophysial joint pain. Spine. 2000;25:1270-7.

7

Sacroiliac Joint Pain

Ari Greis, Melissa Guanche

CHIEF COMPLAINT

The patient complains of right buttock pain.

HISTORY OF PRESENT ILLNESS

A 29-year-old right-handed female presents with an 8-week history of constant achy right buttock pain after a fall at a concert, landing directly on the right buttocks. The pain radiates to her lateral hip and occasionally down her posterior thigh, not past the knee. There is occasional radiation to the right groin. It is worse with sitting and standing, and somewhat relieved with changing positions and anti-inflammatories. She has been unable to run secondary to pain and states that long distance walking has become uncomfortable. She denies any associated bowel or bladder incontinence, unintentional weight loss or weight gain, fever, chills, night sweats, numbness, tingling, or weakness in the lower extremities. She has no history of low back pain, hip pain or known herniated nucleus pulposis.

She is employed as a librarian.

Treatments to date include over the counter nonsteroidal anti-inflammatory medications and acetaminophen with mild relief. She completed 4 weeks of physical therapy with core strengthening and lower limb conditioning with little improvement in pain. She is coming to your office for a more complete understanding of her problem and to explore other options for pain management.

PAST MEDICAL HISTORY

None

PAST SURGICAL HISTORY

Right inguinal hernia repair 10 years ago.

REVIEW OF SYSTEMS

Otherwise negative

FAMILY HISTORY

Parents alive with osteoarthritis, hypothyroidism and hypertension.

SOCIAL HISTORY

One to two glasses of wine most nights of the week, denies smoking, denies illicit drugs.

CURRENT MEDICATIONS

Naprosyn 220 mg twice a day, occasional acetaminophen.

ALLERGIES

None

PHYSICAL EXAMINATION

- *Height*: 5’8”
- *Weight*: 135 lbs
- *Pulse*: 62/minute
- *Blood Pressure*: 110/70 mm Hg
- *Respirations*: 16/minute

General Appearance

Pleasant, cooperative, looks stated age, in no distress.

Gait and tandem gait stable. Romberg sign is negative. Able to heel walk and toe walk without difficulty. Pulses are 2+ in the radial and dorsalis pedis arteries. Babinski testing reveals downgoing toes bilaterally. No palpable step-off in the lumbar spine. No palpable scoliotic curve. No tenderness over the lumbar spinous processes. No lumbar segmental tenderness. No palpable muscle spasm in the lumbar paraspinals. Pain with palpation

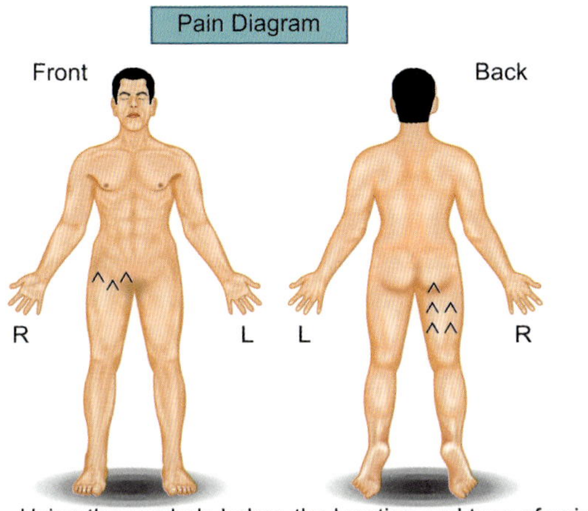

Using the symbols below, the location and type of pain sensations are marked on the diagrams. All the affected areas are included.

TYPE OF SENSATIONS

Aching	^ ^ ^ ^ ^ ^
Sharp or stabbing	X X X X X X
Burning	//////////
Pins and needles	--------------
Numbness	0 0 0 0 0 0

Fig. 7.1: Pain diagram

over the sacral sulcus on the right. No tenderness to palpation over the bilateral trochanteric bursae. Positive "Fortin Finger Test". Slump test and supine straight leg raise to 90° are negative bilaterally. Internal rotation of the hips does not cause pain. No pain with extension or rotation. Negative femoral nerve stretch test bilaterally. Pain in the buttock area with Patrick test on right. Negative Gaenslen's sign, negative Thomas test, negative Ober's test bilaterally. Manual muscle testing in the lower limbs reveals 5/5 bilateral hip flexors, quadriceps, tibialis anterior, extensor hallucis longus, and gastrocsoleus. Sensory examination to light touch and pinprick is normal in the lower extremity dermatomes. Proprioception is intact at the great toes bilaterally. Normal muscle tone. Reflexes are 2+ in patellae, medial hamstrings and Achilles tendons. No ankle clonus bilaterally (Fig. 7.1).

IMAGING

X-rays lumbar spine and pelvis—normal.

Magnetic resonance imaging lumbar spine—minimal bulge at L4-5 without herniated nucleus pulposus or neural compression.

DIAGNOSIS

Sacroiliac Joint Pain

Sacroiliac joint (SIJ) pain is defined as pain localized to the region of the SIJ, reproducible by provocation tests of the SIJ, and reliably relieved by infiltration of the SIJ with a local anesthetic.[1] The prevalence of intra-articular SIJ pain is approximately 10–26.6% in patients with chronic back pain.[2] Its incidence may be overestimated as most studies on the prevalence of SIJ pain focus on patients already suspected of having SIJ pain (pain in the sacral region, SIJ tenderness and positive provocative maneuvers).[3] Manchikanti et al. found the overall incidence of SIJ pain to be only 2% in patients with chronic low back pain.[2] Conversely, some argue it is underestimated as current diagnostic blocks fail to include extra-articular causes (enthesopathy, fractures, ligamentous injuries and myofascial).

The innervation of the SIJ is predominantly dorsal, encompassing a wide range of sensory fiber types from the L5 dorsal ramus and the S1-S4 dorsal rami.[4] Anatomic dissection has illustrated marked variability in the location and number of lateral branch (LB) nerves innervating the dorsal SIJ complex between cadavers and also within individual cadavers.[4] The use of sensory stimulation-guided radiofrequency (RF) to identify symptomatic (pain transmitting) branches demonstrated symptomatic branches stemming predominantly from the L5 dorsal sensory branch (distinct from medial branch of L5 dorsal ramus) and S1 LB, with common symptomatic LBs at S2 and S3.[4] An understanding of the structure and function of the SIJ is necessary in order to successfully design a treatment plan.

The SIJ is a diarthrodial synovial joint that primarily functions as a stress relieving joint for the pelvic ring.[5] It supports the lumbar spine and transmits forces from the vertebral column to the pelvis and lower limbs and vice versa. Its design allows for a small range of movement necessary to counter the torsional stresses encountered with ambulation and postural changes. There are no muscles spcecifically designed to produce active, physiologic movement of the SIJ. Movement occurs passively as a result of muscle contraction at the hip, pelvis and lumbar spine. Consequently, the stability of the SIJ is subject to the integrity of the various SIJ ligaments and surrounding muscle groups. These include the gluteals, hamstrings, hip external rotators, psoas, abdominals, latissimus dorsi, quadratus lumborum and erector spinae.[6]

The biomechanics of the SIJ are complex. The axes of movement of the SIJ have been described to occur in an oblique plane across the pelvis, consistent with its role as a stress-relieving joint.[7] Numerous studies have examined the movements of the SIJ in a variety of postures and movements and found the range of motion is essentially only 1°.[4] Therapeutic manipulation has also been examined and found not to alter joint position.[8]

The presentation of SIJ pain is similar to other causes of low back pain and clinical evaluation requires a thorough musculoskeletal examination of the low back, pelvis, hips, and the lower limbs. Additionally, a full neurologic assessment is necessary to rule out a neurologic source of pain. The most common presenting symptom in patients with SIJ pain is pain or tenderness over the region of the posterior superior iliac spine (PSIS).[9] The "Fortin Finger test" is commonly used as a simple diagnostic aid and is considered positive when the patient points inferomedial to the PSIS within 1 cm, when asked to indicate the region of pain.[9] Pain is commonly described as being unilateral and localized predominantly below the L5 spinous process.[10] A retrospective study conducted to determine the pain referral patterns in patients with injection-confirmed SIJ pain found radiation into the buttock (94%), lower lumbar region (72%), groin (14%) and upper lumbar region (6%).[11] In the same study, 28% of patients experienced pain radiating below the knee.

Radiologic imaging is inconclusive for diagnosing SIJ pain. Plain films can demonstrate degenerative SIJ changes in at least 24.5% of asymptomatic individuals over age 50.[12] No correlation has been consistently demonstrated between imaging findings and injection-confirmed SIJ pain.[13] SIJ imaging is useful in excluding "red flags", but contributes poorly to the diagnosis.

Physical examination maneuvers are designed to either depict asymmetric movement or provoke SIJ pain. The Standing Flexion and Gillet test are commonly used in assessment of the SIJ motion. A study of the standing flexion test demonstrated asymmetric motion in 20% of asymptomatic individuals.[14] Similarly, evaluation of the Gillet test concluded that there was no statistically significant association between it and patients who responded to fluoroscopically guided anesthetic injections.[15]

A number of provocative SIJ maneuvers have been described. The more commonly utilized maneuvers include the distraction test, compression test, thigh thrust test, Patrick maneuver and Gaenslen test. A study from Slipman showed little value in comparing physical examination findings and diagnostic block.[16] Individually, they have weak predictive value, but when used in combination can suggest the diagnosis of SIJ pain. A study comparing the diagnostic accuracy of a multitest regimen of 5 SIJ pain provocation tests with fluoroscopically controlled double SIJ blocks found that when three or more provocation tests are positive, it is probable that the pain is related to the SIJ.[17] Conversely, SIJ pain is less likely if fewer than three tests are positive.[17]

To confirm the diagnosis of SIJ pain, the International Association for the Study of Pain (IASP) criteria mandates that pain should resolve after intra-articular SIJ infiltration with a local anesthetic.[18] The length of time that the pain is relieved also should correspond to the duration of the anesthetic. Controversy exists over the use of a single versus confirmatory (double) second diagnostic block using two different local anesthetics containing different durations of action. A single diagnostic SIJ block has been reported to have a false-positive rate of approximately one-third[12] and studies have found using a double-block paradigm to be more specific and reliable for diagnosing SIJ pain.[15] False-positive blocks may occur secondary to extravasation of local anesthetic to surrounding pain-generating structures such as muscles, ligaments, and lumbosacral nerve roots.[10] Similarly, false-negative blocks may occur with failure to obtain adequate local anesthetic spread to the anterior and cephalad portions of the SIJ.[10] Image-guided needle placement is strongly recommended when performing intra-articular SIJ blocks as one study illustrated only 22% intra-articular injectate spread in blind procedures.[19] Some authors advocate diagnostic dorsal ramus and lateral branch blocks to confirm the diagnosis of SIJ pain.[20]

TREATMENT OPTIONS

Successful treatment of SIJ pain is challenging and best performed in the context of a multidisciplinary approach. Conservative treatments are directed at correcting the underlying biomechanical abnormalities and interventional treatments aim to alleviate symptoms.

Conservative treatment for SIJ pain resulting from postural and gait disturbances include physical therapy and manipulation. Both have been suggested to reduce pain and improve mobility, however, there are no controlled studies evaluating patients with injection-confirmed SIJ pain. Correction of leg length discrepancy with the use of shoe inserts and nonsurgical stabilization with pelvic belts and exercise-induced pelvic stabilization programs are also utilized.[21]

INTERVENTIONAL OPTIONS

Patients with SIJ pain refractory to conservative treatment are candidates for interventional management with intra-articular injections and/or RF treatment.

Intra-articular injections with local anesthetic and steroid can serve the dual function of aiding in confirming the diagnosis and being therapeutic. Studies vary with regard to primary outcome measures and method of diagnosis of SIJ pain, however, most have found image-guided SIJ injections to provide good pain relief lasting from 6 months to 1 year.[10] One study found a significant reduction in Oswestry disability score and visual analog scale pain score (both at the time of discharge from treatment and at almost 2-year follow-up) following one or more therapeutic SIJ injection.

Classical Sacroiliac Joint Infiltration Technique

Informed consent was signed and all the patient's questions were answered. The risks, benefits, and alternative treatment options were explained. The risks include but are not limited to increased pain, superficial or deep

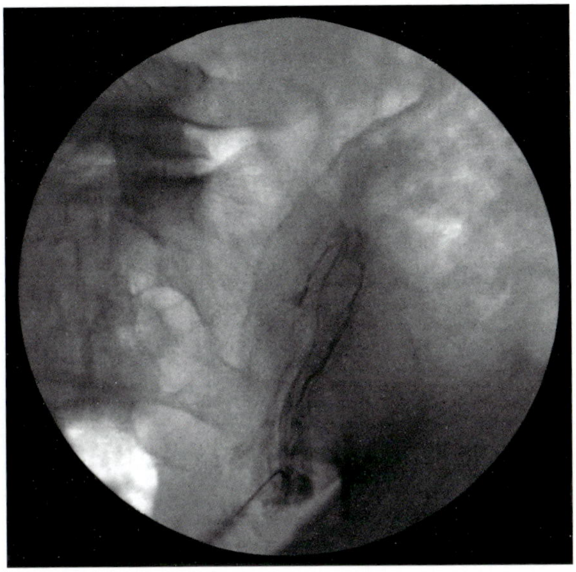

Fig. 7.2: Sacroiliac joint with contrast

infection, allergic reaction, nerve damage, paralysis, syncope, increased blood sugar, headache, respiratory or cardiac arrest, and scar formation. All vital signs, cardiac rhythm and oxygen saturation were monitored prior to, during, and after the procedure.

The C-arm was positioned so that the SIJ was visualized. The soft tissues overlying this structure were infiltrated with a small amount of 1% lidocaine without epinephrine. A 22- or 25-gauge spinal needle was advanced down to the inferior portion of the SIJ and then inserted into the fluoroscopically "hyperlucent" region within the joint. After negative aspirate for blood F, a 0.5–1 cc volume of nonionic contrast was injected and flow of contrast was noted. An injectate consisting of steroid and 1% lidocaine (variable) was administered.

An alternative approach is to visualize the sacroliac joint as medial and lateral projections. This will represent the posterior and anterior aspects of the joint, respectively. The physician will then place the needle into the inferior portion of the medial projection (Fig. 7.2).

Radiofrequency Treatment of the Sacroiliac Joint

Radiofrequency denervation procedures have become increasingly popular over recent years in attempt to provide prolonged pain relief to patients with refractory SIJ pain. There are three main types of radiofrequency ablation (RFA): low-intensity RFA, cooled RFA and pulsed RFA. Studies evaluating

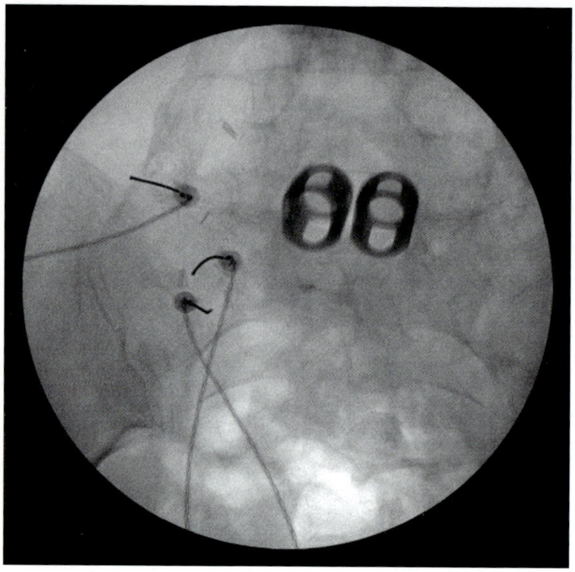

Fig. 7.3: Sacroiliac joint radiofrequency ablation

the use of RFA are limited and differ in the combination of nerves lesioned—no standards have been established for the specific nerves to ablate, type of technique, or type of RFA.[22] The available literature has reported successful outcomes, defined as greater than a 50% consistent decrease in pain, at 6 months[4] and 9 months[22] after the procedure. Newer studies have evaluated "cooled RF", in which electrodes are internally cooled to produce larger thermal lesions and have shown favorable results at 3, 6 and 9 months follow-up.[13,23] There is also literature supporting the use of local anesthetic to the LBs of the sacrum, without intra-articular injection, to determine a good response to SIJ RFA (Fig. 7.3).

Radiofrequency Technique

The patient lies prone and the C-arm is obliqued to view the sacral foramen. An RF lesion generator and an insulated needle with an exposed active tip, either curved or straight is used. The RF needles are placed under fluoroscopic guidance to the regions where the respective nerves supplying the SIJ are known to reside. The electrodes are individually directed under fluoroscopic imaging toward the superior aspect of the sacral ala, approximately 5–7 mm lateral to the S1 superior articular process (location of presumed L5 posterior sensory branch distinct from dorsal ramus medial branch nerve) and the lateral edge of the dorsal sacral foraminal apertures of S1–S3 (sacral dorsal rami LB nerves). At each location, 50 Hz, 1 ms stimulation is applied at 0.4–0.7 V ("searching" voltage). The RF electrodes are finely manipulated under fluoroscopic imaging around the target structures until either reproduction of concordant/usual pain or paresthetic somatic or cutaneous sensation ("benign" stimulation, described by patients as "tingling", "buzzing," or "vibration") is elicited with electrical stimulation. Stimulation is performed through the 2–6 o'clock zone on the right or 6–10 o'clock zone on the left (if the dorsal sacral foramen is viewed as a clock face). If the patient experiences precise reproduction of concordant ipsilateral pain, stimulation voltage is decreased to a threshold of 0.1–0.2 V and the electrodes are finely maneuvered to maximize and maintain stimulation at the minimal threshold voltage. This is also utilized to confirm no radicular sensory stimulation. Motor stimulation may be utilized to ensure that there is no radicular spread of current at 2 Hz. Before RF lesioning, 0.5–1.0 mL of lidocaine is injected to anesthetize the target area. A single LB RF lesion is created at each level (L5, S1, S2). RF lesions are created at 80°C for a period of 60–90 seconds. Lesions are normally repeated one to two times for an additional 60–90 seconds with some slight repositioning of the RF needles. This is to allow for a more complete lesion. Some practitioners may elect to place an alequot of steroid and anesthetic at the end of the case to reduce local inflammation created by the lesioning procedure.

Potential complications can be site soreness, local hematoma, cellulitis, or inadvertent lesioning of a radicular nerve.[24]

REFERENCES

1. Vanelderen P, Szadek K, Cohen SP, et al. 13. Sacroiliac joint pain. Pain Pract. 2010;10(5):470-8.
2. Manchikanti L, Singh V, Pampati V, et al. Evaluation of the relative contributions of various structures in chronic low back pain. Pain Physician. 2001;4(4):308-16.
3. Hansen HC, McKenzie-Brown AM, Cohen SP, et al. Sacroiliac joint interventions: a systematic review. Pain Physician. 2007;10(1):165-184.
4. Yin W, Willard F, Carreiro J, et al. Sensory stimulation-guided sacroiliac joint radiofrequency neurotomy: technique based on neuroanatomy of the dorsal sacral plexus. Spine. 2003;28(20):2419-25.
5. Bogduk N. Clinical and radiological anatomy of the lumbar spine, 5th edition. Philadelphia; 2012.
6. Prather H, Hunt D. Conservative management of low back pain, part I. Sacroiliac joint pain. Dis Mon. 2004;50(12):670-83.
7. Lavignolle B, Vital JM, Senegas J, et al. An approach to the functional anatomy of the sacroiliac joints in vivo. Anat Clin. 1983;5(3):169-76.
8. Tullberg T, Blomberg S, Branth B, et al. Manipulation does not alter the position of the sacroiliac joint. A roentgen stereophotogrammetric analysis. Spine. 1998;23(10):1124-8; discussion 1129.
9. Fortin JD, Falco FJ. The Fortin finger test: an indicator of sacroiliac pain. Am J Orthop. 1997; 26(7):477-80.
10. Cohen SP. Sacroiliac joint pain: a comprehensive review of anatomy, diagnosis, and treatment. Anesth Analg. 2005;101(5):1440-53.
11. Slipman CW, Jackson HB, Lipetz JS, et al. Sacroiliac joint pain referral zones. Arch Phys Med Rehabil. 2000;81(3):334-8.

12. Chou LH, Slipman CW, Bhagia SM, et al. Inciting events initiating injection-proven sacroiliac joint syndrome. Pain Medicine. 2004;5(1):26-32.
13. Patel N, Gross A, Brown L, et al. A randomized, placebo-controlled study to assess the efficacy of lateral branch neurotomy for chronic sacroiliac joint pain. Pain Med. 2012;13(3):383-98.
14. Dreyfuss P, Dryer S, Griffin J, et al. Positive sacroiliac screening tests in asymptomatic adults. Spine. 1994;19(10):1138-43.
15. Maigne JY, Aivaliklis A, Pfefer F. Results of sacroiliac joint double block and value of sacroiliac pain provocation tests in 54 patients with low back pain. Spine. 1996;21(6):1889-92.
16. Slipman CW, Sterenfeld EB, Chou LH, et al. The predictive value of provocative sacroiliac joint stress maneuvers in the diagnosis of sacroiliac joint syndrome. Arch Phys Med Rehabil. 1998;79(3):288-92.
17. van der Wurff P, Buijs EJ, Groen GJ. A multitest regimen of pain provocation tests as an aid to reduce unnecessary minimally invasive sacroiliac joint procedures. Arch Phys Med Rehabil. 2006;87(1):10-4.
18. Merskey H, Bogduk N (Eds). Chronic pain: descriptions of chronic pain syndromes and definitions of pain terms, 2nd edition. Seattle, WA: IASP Press; 1994. pp. 39-43.
19. Rosenberg JM, Quint TJ, de Rosayro AM. Computerized tomographic localization of clinically-guided sacroiliac joint injections. Clin J Pain. 2000;16(1):18-21.
20. Cohen SP, Abdi S. Lateral branch blocks as a treatment for sacroiliac joint pain: A pilot study. Reg Anesth Pain Med. 2003;28(2):113-9.
21. Mooney V, Pozos R, Vleeming A, et al. Exercise treatment for sacroiliac pain. Orthopedics. 2001; 24(1):29-32.
22. Aydin SM, Gharibo CG, Mehnert M, et al. The role of radiofrequency ablation for sacroiliac joint pain: a meta-analysis. PM & R. 2010;2(9):842-51.
23. Cheng J, Pope JE, Dalton JE, et al. Comparative outcomes of cooled versus traditional radiofrequency ablation of the lateral branches for sacroiliac joint pain. Clin J Pain. 2013;29(2):132-7.
24. Abbott Z, Smuck M, Haig A, et al. Irreversible spinal nerve injury from dorsal ramus radiofrequency neurotomy: a case report. Arch Phys Med Rehabil. 2007;88(10):1350-2.

8

Cervical Disc Herniation with Radiculopathy

Theodore Conliffe, Jeremy Simon, Zachary Broyer

CHIEF COMPLAINT

The patient complains of neck and left arm pain.

HISTORY OF PRESENT ILLNESS

The patient is a 33-year-old right-hand dominant professional football player who presented to our office with a chief complaint of neck pain radiating into his left arm for approximately 4 weeks. His injury occurred while making a tackle on a running back during practice. He tackled the ball carrier with his left shoulder and violently drove the player to the ground. He initially was without discomfort but developed a burning ache in his neck and left shoulder over the next few days. His symptoms have persisted despite use of nonsteroidal anti-inflammatory drugs, heat and ice by his trainers. He has also tried to remedy his symptoms with therapeutic massage and chiropractic adjustments without benefit thus far.

The patient informed our staff that he had a similar episode about 3 years ago and frequently complains of neck stiffness and soreness after games. He recalls one episode that his entire left arm went numb for about 5 minutes and he was told that he had a "stinger" but the symptoms resolved quickly without further incident.

The patient describes his current symptoms as a constant dull ache in his neck with associated pain in his left shoulder and scapula with numbness into his left hand (Fig. 8.1). He quantifies his level of pain as a 7/10 on a visual analog scale. The symptoms are not accompanied by motor weakness, clumsiness, or loss of control of bowel or bladder. There is no balance or fine motor deficits. The symptoms are exacerbated by neck flexion and lateral

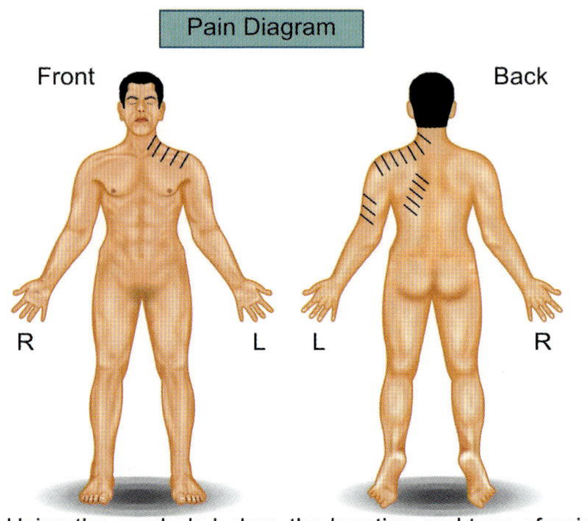

Using the symbols below, the location and type of pain sensations are marked on the diagrams. All the affected areas are included.

TYPE OF SENSATIONS

Aching	^ ^ ^ ^ ^ ^
Sharp or stabbing	X X X X X X
Burning	//////////
Pins and needles	---------------
Numbness	0 0 0 0 0 0

Fig. 8.1: Pain diagram

flexion of his neck to his right shoulder, as well as reaching overhead. His symptoms are not relieved by anything presently.

PAST MEDICAL HISTORY

Cervical strain, right shoulder dislocation.

PAST SURGICAL HISTORY

Right anterior cruciate ligament reconstruction, left meniscectomy.

FAMILY HISTORY

Unremarkable

MEDICATIONS

Ibuprofen 600 mg taken with food, metaxalone (skelaxin) 800 mg QHS.

ALLERGIES

Penicillin

SOCIAL HISTORY

Patient is a nonsmoker. Drinks alcohol socially.

REVIEW OF SYSTEMS

Neck pain, left arm pain/numbness.

PHYSICAL EXAMINATION

Vital Signs

- *Height*: 6' 2"
- *Weight*: 225 lbs
- *Pulse*: 56/minute
- *Blood pressure*: 120/74 mm Hg

General Appearance

Well-developed, well-nourished male in no apparent distress at time of examination.

The patient's gait and station are normal and his coordination is intact for rapid alternating movements. Inspection and palpation revealed *tenderness over the left cervical paraspinal muscles and trapezius.*

Motor strength was normal and 5/5 in all extremities. *There was mildly diminished sensation to light touch in the first digit of the left hand.*

Reflexes

Left biceps reflex was 1 + otherwise, all other reflexes were intact. There were no upper motor neuron signs, including Hoffman's and Babinski signs.

Provocative tests: *Spurling's maneuver was positive for reproduction of pain into his left arm.*

Range of motion was normal in flexion/extension and lateral rotation of C-spine, however, *pain was reproduced with neck flexion past 10°.*

There were normal movements observed in the patient's shoulders, hips and knees. There were negative provocative maneuvers for shoulder pain.

No other abnormalities were observed on physical examination.

IMAGING STUDIES

X-Rays

Anteroposterior, lateral, flexion and extension X-rays of cervical spine were obtained and revealed moderate cervical spondylosis with narrowing of the cervical zygapophyseal joints bilaterally from C4 to C7. There was no spondylolisthesis, fracture or instability observed with dynamic imaging.

Magnetic Resonance Imaging

Magnetic resonance imaging (MRI) of the cervical spine revealed a *moderate broad-based disc osteophyte complex at C5/6 with mild narrowing of the neuroforamen on the left.* There was no spinal cord impingement or signal changes within the spinal cord. All other levels had mild degenerative changes without significant neural encroachment.

DIAGNOSIS

Cervical disc herniation with left C6 radiculopathy.

TREATMENT OPTIONS

The patient's occupation as a professional football player requires that he returns to play as soon as possible without missing any games necessitating a fairly aggressive approach.

The patient was receiving physical therapy with emphasis on cervical stabilization exercises as prescribed by his team physicians and training staff.

He referred himself to a local chiropractor for adjustments and received four to six sessions without benefit, and this treatment could be continued. While not conclusive, some data suggests that manipulation in disorders of the cervical spine may be beneficial.[1,2] Complications with manipulation are rare, but reported.[3-9] Cervical traction can be considered as an adjunctive, nonmedication, noninvasive treatment. Studies on its benefit are conflicting.[10-12]

Medication options include nonsteroidal anti-inflammatories, muscle relaxants and/or membrane stabilizing medications. Opiates in the setting of radiculopathy should not be considered as a first line agent. This patient declined additional medications.

The patient also had the option of therapeutic massage and electrical stimulation that may provide some benefits with this condition. The studies on these modalities are also conflicting.[13,14] In addition, there are currently no well-controlled randomized controlled studies proving the benefits of massage therapy in neck pain or cervical radiculopathy.[15]

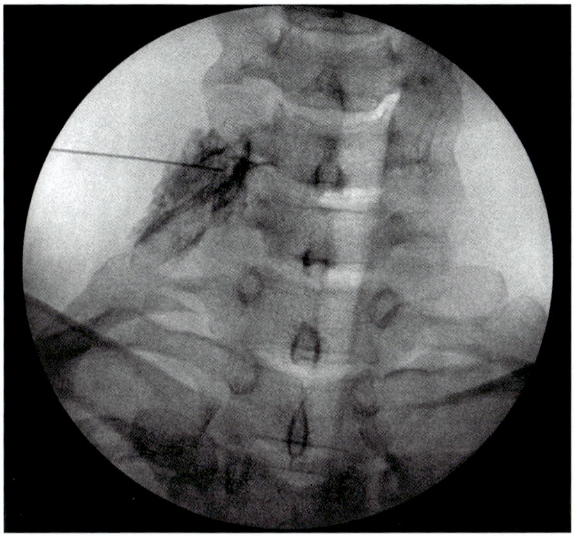

Fig. 8.2: Left cervical transforaminal epidural steroid injection

At the time of his evaluation it was too soon to consider surgical intervention and this option would have ended the patient's season. The absence of progressive neurologic dysfunction or overt signs of myelopathy allow for nonsurgical management. The indications for cervical spine surgery include but are not limited to progressive neurological deficits, intractable arm pain, loss of bladder or bowel function, and other symptoms and signs of myelopathy.[16,17] The absence of cord edema and severe cord impingement allow for the consideration of a cervical epidural steroid injection (Fig. 8.2).

The decision was made to proceed with a cervical transforaminal epidural steroid injection targeting the C6 nerve root on the left.

INDICATIONS

Pain radiates into the left upper extremity corresponding to the cervical symptoms of C6 radiculopathy. A cervical MRI prior to considering the procedure supported the diagnosis. The patient attempted to control his symptoms with 4 weeks of conservative treatments including physical therapy, medications and chiropractic manipulations without success.

The patient's symptoms of predominant arm versus neck pain made us choose a transforaminal versus interlaminar approach, although there is no definitive evidence that one approach is superior to the other.[18,19]

Cervical Epidural Steroid Injection: Transforaminal Approach

Following informed consent the patient was brought to the fluoroscopy suite and placed in the supine position. An intravenous catheter was inserted into the patient forearm for administration of fluids and mild conscious sedation.

The patient's neck was sterilely prepped and draped in the usual fashion. C-arm fluoroscope was positioned in the oblique position to identify the neuroforamen of the targeted nerve root (Left C6). The target position is the posterior aspect of the cervical intervertebral foramen of the exiting spinal nerve. A sterile spinal needle is directed through the skin over the target and the needle is inserted using the axis of the fluoroscope into the posterior aspect of the intervertebral foramen. Needle positioning is confirmed by oblique view demonstration of needle placement in the posterior aspect of the foremen and anterior posterior view lateral placement of the needle.

Confirmation of the needle placement in the epidural space is made by injection of 1.0 cc of iodinated contrast. Live fluoroscopic images are obtained in the anterior posterior view to confirm placement of contrast spread along the nerve root and to ensure no vascular spread specifically within the vertebral artery.

After needle placement is confirmed 1–2 cc of preservative-free 1% lidocaine is injected and the patient is monitored briefly to ensure no seizure activity. Finally, 1 cc of corticosteroid, dexamethasone equivalent to 10 mg, is injected and the needle is removed.

The patient is then taken to the recovery room and monitored for approximately 30 minutes to 1 hour prior to discharge. The patient is provided with discharge instructions about contacting the physician after the procedure and follow-up appointments are scheduled.

DISCUSSION

The proposed theory behind epidural steroid injection is that the corticosteroids diminish inflammation caused by the disc herniation. Saal et al. described high levels of inflammatory phospholipase A2 in lumbar disc herniation.[20]

Cervical epidural steroid injections were first described in medical literature in the 1960s to treat radiculopathy.[21] Since that time, these procedures have become a widespread treatment for cervical radiculopathy. The evidence supporting efficacy of epidural steroid injections is limited by the absence of randomized controlled trials.

Slipman et al.[22] retrospectively analyzed selective nerve root blocks in scientific literature for the cervical spine and reported there were clear benefits and improved pain control. The evidence surrounding efficacy of cervical epidural steroid injections for axial neck pain is limited. A recent small randomized controlled study by Manchikanti et al. in 2010 for discogenic neck pain showed benefits of pain relief and improved functional status.[23]

A retrospective analysis by Benyamin et al. found there to be moderate evidence that cervical interlaminar epidural injections provided relief of chronic neck and radicular pain.[24] Presently, there is some controversy regarding the application of cervical transforaminal epidural steroids in the use of radicular pain. The relative safety of these procedures has been debated due to the potential for catastrophic injury. The potential for paralysis, stroke and death exists by accidental injection into a vertebral artery despite fluoroscopic imaging in expert hands.[25-27] Many clinicians have stopped performing these procedures because of the risk and instead perform only cervical interlaminar injections.

CLINICAL OUTCOME

The patient received a left C6 transforaminal epidural injection without complications and was able to return to practice and play in the game within a week of his injection. Thus far he has avoided further injury to his cervical spine and hopes to avoid surgical intervention in the future.

REFERENCES

1. Eriksen K, Rochester RP, Hurwitz EL. Symptomatic reactions, clinical outcomes and patient satisfaction associated with upper cervical chiropractic care: a prospective, multicenter, cohort study. BMC Musculoskeletal Disorders. 2011;12:219.
2. Hurwitz EL, Aker PD, Adams AH, et al. Manipulation and mobilization of the cervical spine. A systematic review of the literature. Spine. 1996; 21(15):1746-59; discussion 1759-60.
3. Lopez-Gonzalez A, Peris-Celda M. Acute paraplegia after chiropraxis. European spine journal: official publication of the European Spine Society, the European Spinal Deformity Society, and the European Section of the Cervical Spine Research Society. 2011;20 (Suppl 2):S143-6.
4. Chakraverty J, Curtis O, Hughes T, et al. Spinal cord injury following chiropractic manipulation to the neck. Acta Radiol. 2011;52(10):1125-7.
5. Solheim O, Jorgensen JV, Nygaard OP. Lumbar epidural hematoma after chiropractic manipulation for lower-back pain: case report. Neurosurgery. 2007;61(1):E170-1; discussion E171.
6. Whedon JM. Lumbar epidural hematoma after chiropractic manipulation for lower-back pain: case report. Neurosurgery 2008;63(2):E376; author reply E376.
7. Soragna D, Montalbetti L, Bo P, et al. Chiropractic complications. Another case report. Acta Neurol. 1993;15(2):145-50.
8. Stuart PJ, Bernstein T. A case of subdural hematoma and temporal bone fracture as complications of chiropractic manipulation. J Emerg Med. 1989;7(6):615-7.
9. Huff L. Chiropractic manipulation and incidence of complications. Am Fam Physician. 1996; 54(5):1467, 1470.
10. Zylbergold RS, Piper MC. Cervical spine disorders. A comparison of three types of traction. Spine. 1985;10(10):867-71.

11. Ellenberg MR, Honet JC, Treanor WJ. Cervical radiculopathy. Arch Phy Med Rehabil. 1994; 75(3):342-52.
12. Thoomes EJ, Scholten-Peeters W, Koes B, et al. The Effectiveness of Conservative Treatment for Patients with Cervical Radiculopathy: A Systematic Review. Clin J Pain. 2013.
13. Chiu TT, Hui-Chan CW, Chein G. A randomized clinical trial of TENS and exercise for patients with chronic neck pain. Clinical Rehabil. 2005; 19(8): 850-60.
14. Frieden RA. Conservative management of neck pain. Mt Sinai J Medicine. 1994;61(3):197-203.
15. Gam AN, Warming S, Larsen LH, et al. Treatment of myofascial trigger-points with ultrasound combined with massage and exercise—a randomised controlled trial. Pain. 1998;77(1):73-9.
16. Nesterenko SO, Riley LH, Skolasky RL. Anterior cervical discectomy and fusion versus cervical disc arthroplasty: current state and trends in treatment for cervical disc pathology. Spine. 2012; 37(17):1470-4.
17. Dreyer SJ, Boden SD. Nonoperative treatment of neck and arm pain. Spine. 1998;23(24):2746-54.
18. Smuck M, Rosenberg JM, Akuthota V. The use of epidural corticosteroids for cervical radiculopathy: an interlaminar versus transforaminal approach. PM R. 2009;1(2):178-84.
19. Diwan S, Manchikanti L, Benyamin RM, et al. Effectiveness of cervical epidural injections in the management of chronic neck and upper extremity pain. Pain Physician. 2012;15(4):E405-34.
20. Saal JS, Franson RC, Dobrow R, et al. High levels of inflammatory phospholipase A2 activity in lumbar disc herniations. Spine. 1990;15(7):674-8.
21. Thierry-Mieg J. [Cervical epidural injections of corticoids in hyperalgic cervico-brachial neuralgias. 1st cervical epidurographical pictures]. Rev Rhum Mal Osteoartic. 1961;28:451-3.
22. Slipman CW, Lipetz JS, Jackson HB, et al. Therapeutic selective nerve root block in the nonsurgical treatment of atraumatic cervical spondylotic radicular pain: a retrospective analysis with independent clinical review. Arch Phy Med Rehabil. 2000;81(6):741-6.
23. Manchikanti L, Cash KA, Pampati V, et al. Cervical epidural injections in chronic discogenic neck pain without disc herniation or radiculitis: preliminary results of a randomized, double-blind, controlled trial. Pain Physician. 2010;13(4): E265-78.
24. Benyamin RM, Singh V, Parr AT, et al. Systematic review of the effectiveness of cervical epidurals in the management of chronic neck pain. Pain Physician. 2009;12(1):137-57.
25. Huston CW, Slipman CW, Garvin C. Complications and side effects of cervical and lumbosacral selective nerve root injections. Arch Phy Med Rehabil. 2005;86(2):277-83.
26. Scanlon GC, Moeller-Bertram T, Romanowsky SM, et al. Cervical transforaminal epidural steroid injections: more dangerous than we think? Spine. 2007;32(11): 1249-56.
27. Rozin L, Rozin R, Koehler SA, et al. Death during transforaminal epidural steroid nerve root block (C7) due to perforation of the left vertebral artery. Am J Forensic Med Pathol. 2003;24(4):351-5.

9

Cervical Disc Herniation without Radiculopathy

Gautam Kothari, Jeremy Simon

CHIEF COMPLAINT

The patient complains of neck pain.

HISTORY OF PRESENT ILLNESS

A 39-year-old gentleman with a 3-year-history of intermittent axial neck pain presents with 6 months of worsening symptoms. He describes symptom exacerbation after going to an amusement park and going on multiple rollercoaster rides. He noted that a week following the rides, he began experiencing worsening neck pain which was associated with spasm (Fig. 9.1). The symptoms are also described as "sharp and burning" and are exacerbated by prolonged neck flexion/extension and rotation, which is a requirement of his job as an electrician. He has no significant history of neck pain or radiating arm pain. His pain level is currently an 8/10. He does not describe any associated falling, fine-motor deficits, clumsiness, loss of bowel or bladder control, or any other constitutional symptoms.

Treatments to date have been conservative and include 6 weeks of physical therapy to the cervical spine including stabilization, range of motion exercises, modalities with cervical traction and strengthening of the upper extremities and paraspinal musculature. He was given a Medrol Dosepak initially and has been more recently been taking nonsteroidal anti-inflammatory medications twice daily and a muscle relaxer at night time for sleep and spasm. His primary care physician recently started him on tramadol for his pain. He has noticed minimal relief with these treatments. He has also tried a few chiropractic treatments with no significant benefit.

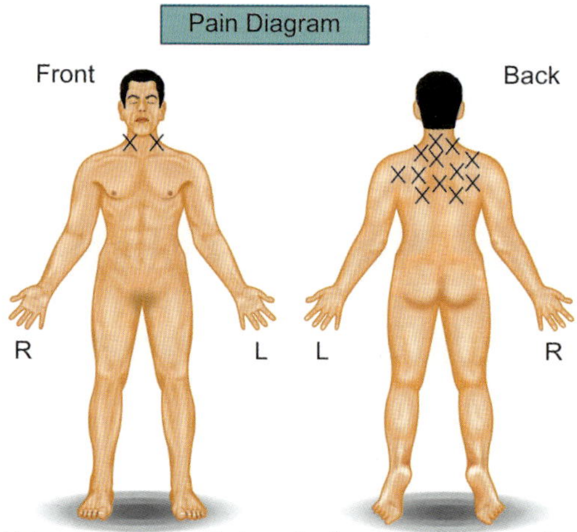

Using the symbols below, the location and type of pain sensations are marked on the diagrams. All the affected areas are included.

TYPE OF SENSATIONS

Aching	^ ^ ^ ^ ^ ^
Sharp or stabbing	X X X X X X
Burning	//////////
Pins and needles	---------------
Numbness	0 0 0 0 0 0

Fig. 9.1: Pain diagram

He is presenting to your office for a more complete evaluation of his problem and to explore the possibility of spinal intervention. He brings with him a recent cervical spine MRI ordered by his primary care physician.

PAST MEDICAL/SURGICAL HISTORY

None

FAMILY HISTORY

Parents alive, both healthy.

SOCIAL HISTORY

Currently employed as an electrician, drinks: two drinks/week, denies tobacco, denies illicit drug use, no workman's compensation claim or autoclaim.

MEDICATIONS

Ibuprofen 800 mg PO TID PRN, cyclobenzaprine 10 mg PO QHS PRN, tramadol 50 mg PO BID PRN.

ALLERGIES

None

REVIEW OF SYSTEMS

Negative

PHYSICAL EXAMINATION

- *Height*: 5'7"
- *Weight*: 175
- *Pulse*: 80/minute
- *Respirations*: 16/minute

General Appearance

Pleasant, cooperative, looks stated age in no acute distress.

Affect is unremarkable. Coordination is normal. Reflexes are 2/4 right biceps, triceps and brachioradialis. *Left biceps and brachioradialis are 1/4 and left triceps at 2/4*. Hoffmann is negative. Inspection and palpation do not identify significant misalignment, atrophy, or asymmetry in the head, neck, shoulders, upper limbs or thoracolumbar spine. There is no evidence of acute dislocation, instability or fracture in the neck, thoracolumbar spine or either upper limb. The pelvis is level without obvious scoliotic deformity. The patient has a normal tandem gait. *Cervical flexion and extension are painful, rotation and side bending to the left side also painful*, pain free toward the right. *Spurling's maneuver reproduces left axial neck pain*. Bilateral shoulder forward flexion, abduction, internal and external rotation range of motion is grossly functional and symmetric. Strength testing is 5/5 in the right upper extremity. Left upper extremity strength demonstrates 5/5 muscle strength testing with the exception of *left elbow flexion and wrist extension which is 4/5*. *Sensation* to light touch is normal in the right upper extremity, diminished in the *left proximal outer arm and distal radial forearm*. Distal pulses are within normal limits in the bilateral upper limbs, neck and trunk without evidence of lymphadenopathy, edema, or rash in these regions. There is no ankle clonus.

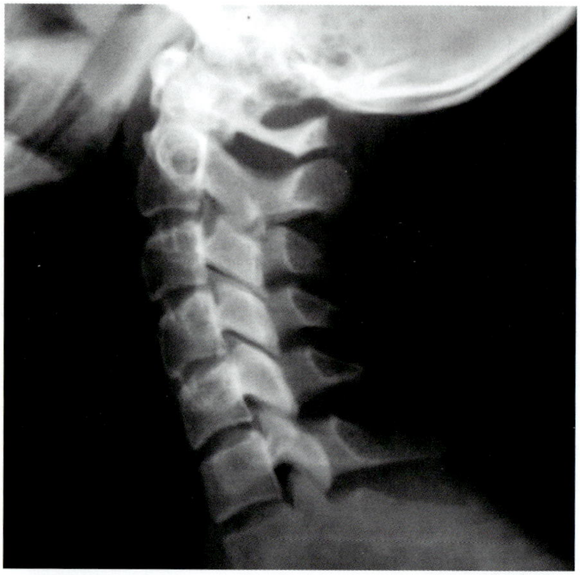

Fig. 9.2: Lateral radiograph of the cervical spine

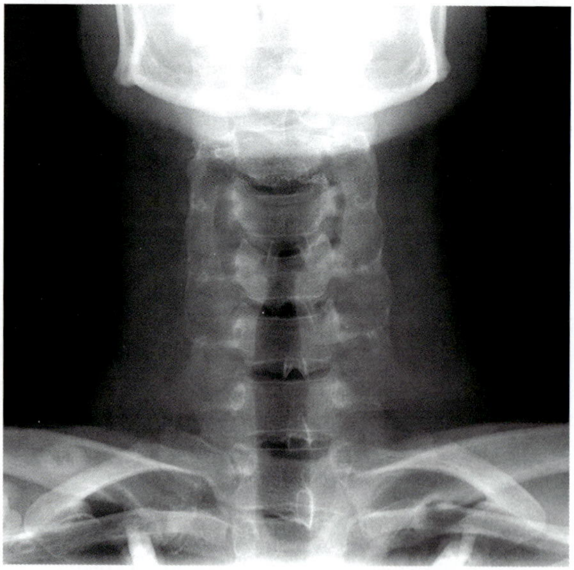

Fig. 9.3: Anterior-posterior (AP) radiograph of the cervical spine

IMAGING

X-ray cervical spine (anteroposterior/Lat/obl/flex/ext) demonstrated normal alignment and contour (Figs 9.2 to 9.4). Reduced lordosis. No instability on flexion/extension. No evidence of fracture or dislocation. No evidence of spondylolisthesis.

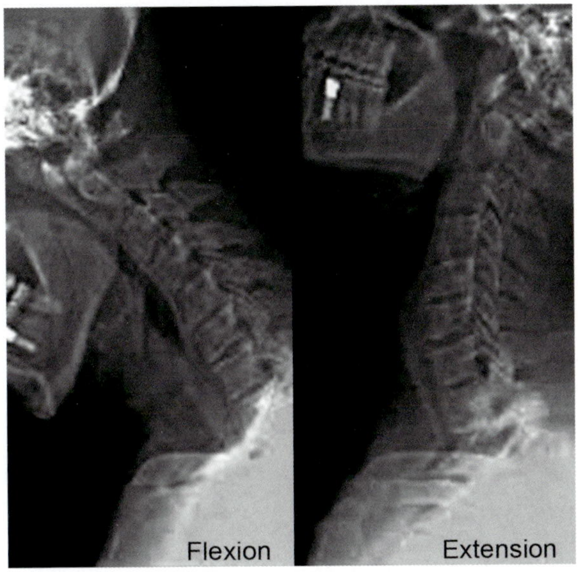

Fig. 9.4: Lateral flexion-extension radiographs of the cervical spine

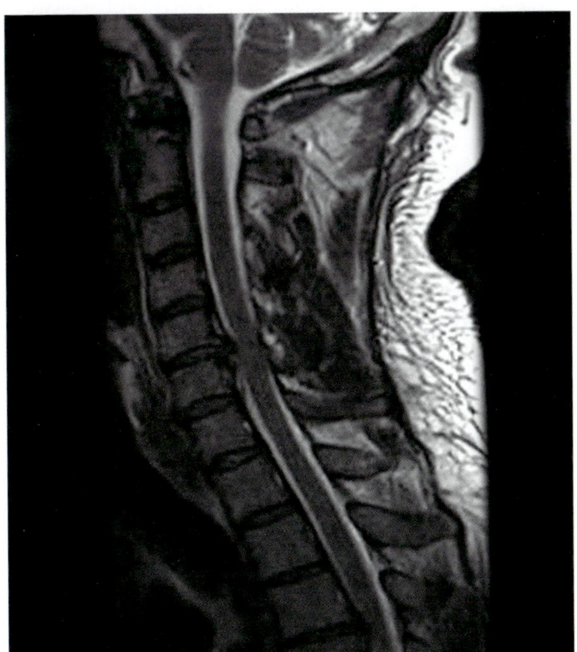

Fig. 9.5: Sagittal MRI showing a C5-6 disc herniation

Magnetic imaging of the cervical spine without contrast demonstrates a moderate-sized central disc herniation at C5–C6 with effacement of the ventral aspect of the spinal cord (Fig. 9.5).

DIAGNOSIS

Axial neck pain in the setting of cervical disc herniation C5–C6.

TREATMENT OPTIONS

The patient presents with axial neck pain appearing to be largely discogenic in nature. His symptoms have been minimally responsive to physical therapy, manual therapies, and medication management. Consideration should certainly be given to continuation of cervical spine stabilization and strengthening as the patient's job requires a significant amount of cervical flexion/extension.

The patient is currently on ibuprofen 800 MG PO TID as well as cyclobenzaprine and tramadol. Although the patient is otherwise healthy, he should be counseled with regards to long-term effects of anti-inflammatory medications and should certainly have a H2 blocker or proton pump inhibitor added to his regimen for gastric protection.[1] The dosage of tramadol could be increased, but a frank discussion is necessary regarding the addiction and tolerance potential of this drug.[2]

The symptoms, physical exam findings and imaging studies correlate with a discogenic neck pain. Cervical facet syndrome is less likely as he does not have evidence of cervical facet disease on imaging.

INTERVENTIONAL OPTIONS

Axial neck pain has a typical 12-month prevalence of 30–50%.[3] In recent years chronic neck pain has reached epidemic proportions with an explosion in diagnostic and therapeutic measures. There is, to date, no consensus on the cause and/or treatment. The pain generators can range from soft tissue to symptomatic facet disease to symptomatic discogenic pain. It has been postulated that the presence of discogenic pain can be wide ranging because of the multi-segmental innervation of the intervertebral disc. Dorsal root ganglia, sympathetic ganglia and parasympathetic ganglia can all contribute to innervation of the disc. This may explain the prevalence of discogenic pain that can occur via different arms of the nervous system.[4] Advanced diagnostic imaging offers an anatomic road map of degenerative disc disease and potential pain generators, but does not necessarily correlate with subjective complaints. For this reason, patients with recalcitrant axial neck pain who have not responded to conservative management may be candidates for diagnostic discography.[5] Serious complications including discitis can occur[6] and the true utility of the procedure is in question.[7]

Cervical epidural steroid injections can be considered for the treatment of axial neck pain in the setting of a disc herniation not responding well to other conservative measures.[3] The proposed mechanism of epidural steroid injections is a reduction in axial and radicular pain by administration of a concentrated mixture of localized steroid/anesthetic in close proximity to the site of pathology, thereby reducing the inflammatory reaction likely responsible for symptoms. The efficacy of epidurals is considered greater in those patients with radicular pain, in the presence of disc herniation or stenosis, and is less predictable for patients with axial pain without radicular symptoms with similar anatomic abnormalities.[8]

The approach that is commonly considered is through the interlaminar approach (Figs 9.6 to 9.8). This procedure is carried out with the use of fluoroscopic guidance. The target entry point is (generally) the C7–T1 interspace as this is considered the safest entry point. It has the largest epidural space relative to the dura and spinal cord in the cervical spine thereby allowing more room to work.[9] Similar to lumbar interlaminar injections, the paramedian approach is what is most commonly used to avoid traversing the interspinous ligament. Biplanar imaging is advocated for safe needle placement and assessment of depth of needle insertion. Commonly, the patient's shoulders obscure the needle image on lateral view. In this scenario, the 60° contralateral oblique view may be the only view available for safely identifying depth. If the needle tip is midline, the oblique may be in either direction (i.e. right or left). When the lateral or contralateral view is used, "stepping off" lamina is not necessary.[10,11]

Cervical Interlaminar Epidural Steroid Injections

The patient was prepped and draped in a sterile fashion in the prone position after informed consent was signed and all patient questions were answered

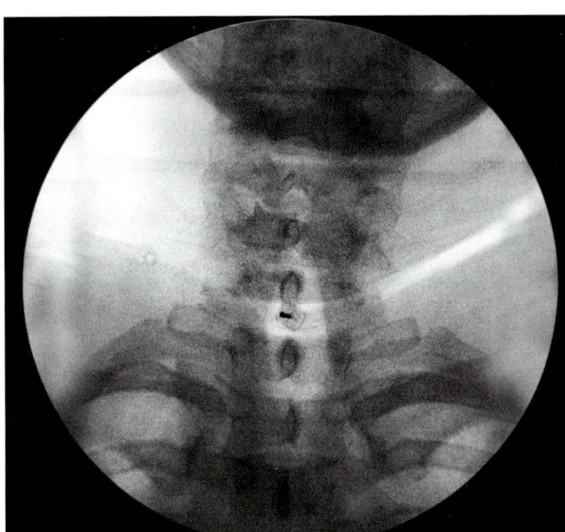

Fig. 9.6: AP fluoroscopy image showing the Tuohy needle in the C7-T1 interspace

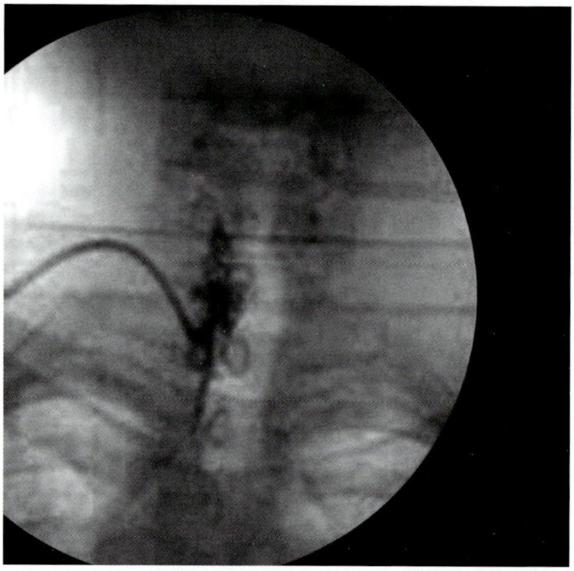

Fig. 9.7: AP fluoroscopy image showing the flow of contrast epidurally and lateralizing to the left

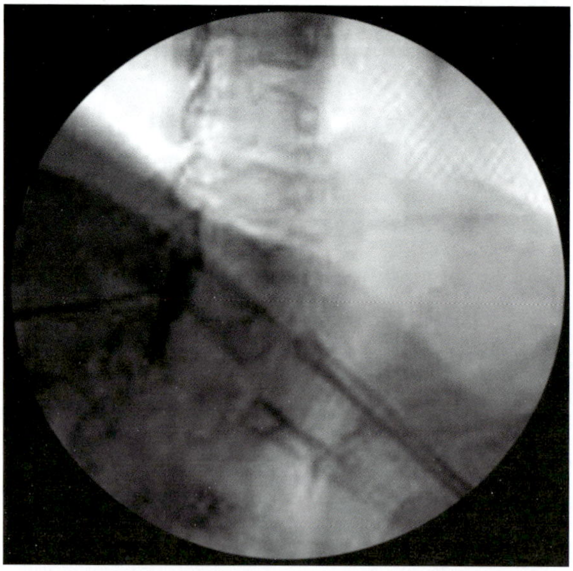

Fig. 9.8: Contralateral oblique image showing the flow of contrast into the epidural space

including the risks, benefits, alternative treatment options and prognosis. The risks include but are not limited to infection, allergic reaction, nerve damage, stroke, paralysis, epidural hematoma, syncope, headache, respiratory or cardiac arrest, spinal cord injury, and scar formation.

Using a paramedian approach from the side mentioned above, the region overlying the inferior lamina was localized under fluoroscopic visualization and the soft tissues overlying this structure were infiltrated with 4 cc. of 1% lidocaine without epinephrine. A #18 gauge, Tuohy needle was inserted into the epidural space using a paramedian approach. The epidural space was localized using loss of resistance after negative aspirate for air, blood, and CSF. A 2 cc volume of omnipaque 300 was injected into the epidural space and the flow of contrast was observed. Radiographs were obtained for documentation purposes.

The injectate was administered into the level noted above. The patient tolerated the procedure well and was discharged after an appropriate period of observation.

If there are any complications, the patient was instructed to call us.

The patient is to follow-up with the requesting physician in 1–2 weeks.

REFERENCES

1. Taha AS, Hudson N, Hawkey CJ, et al. Famotidine for the prevention of gastric and duodenal ulcers caused by nonsteroidal antiinflammatory drugs. N Engl J Med. 1996;334(22):1435-9.
2. Raffa RB, Friderichs E, Reimann W, et al. Complementary and synergistic antinociceptive interaction between the enantiomers of tramadol. J Pharmacol Exp Ther. 1993;267(1):331-40.
3. Manchikanti L, Cash KA, Pampati V, et al. Cervical epidural injections in chronic discogenic neck pain without disc herniation or radiculitis: preliminary results of a randomized, double-blind, controlled trial. Pain physician. 2010; 13(4): E265-78.
4. Fujimoto K, Miyagi M, Ishikawa T, et al. Sensory and autonomic innervation of the cervical intervertebral disc in rats: the pathomechanics of chronic discogenic neck pain. Spine. 2012; 37(16):1357-62.
5. Schellhas KP, Smith MD, Gundry CR, et al. Cervical discogenic pain. Prospective correlation of magnetic resonance imaging and discography in asymptomatic subjects and pain sufferers. Spine. 1996;21(3):300-11; discussion 311-2.
6. Kapoor SG, Huff J, Cohen SP. Systematic review of the incidence of discitis after cervical discography. Spine J. 2010;10(8):739-45.
7. Onyewu O, Manchikanti L, Falco FJ, et al. An update of the appraisal of the accuracy and utility of cervical discography in chronic neck pain. Pain Physician. 2012;15(6):E777-806.
8. Bush K, Hillier S. Outcome of cervical radiculopathy treated with periradicular/epidural corticosteroid injections: a prospective study with independent clinical review. European spine journal: official publication of the European Spine Society, the European Spinal Deformity Society, and the European Section of the Cervical Spine Research Society. 1996;5:319-25.
9. Lieberman R, Dreyfuss P, Baker R. Fluoroscopically guided interlaminar cervical epidural injections. Arch Phy Med Rehabil. 2003;84:1568-9; author reply 1569.
10. Furman M, Jasper NR, Lin HW. Fluoroscopic contralateral oblique view in interlaminar interventions: a technical note. Pain Med. 2012; 13(11):1389-96.
11. Landers MH, Dreyfuss P, Bogduk N. On the geometry of fluoroscopy views for cervical interlaminar epidural injections. Pain Med. 2012;13(1):58-65.

10

Cervical Facet Syndrome

Matthew McAuliffe, Jeremy Simon

CHIEF COMPLAINT

The patient complains of neck pain.

HISTORY OF PRESENT ILLNESS

A 37-year-old right-handed male with a 2-year history of neck pain presents to your office. Onset began immediately after he was in a motor vehicle accident where he was a restrained passenger in a rear-end collision. The pain has been a constant dull ache since the accident, worsening over the last 2 weeks. The pain limits his neck motion when looking to the right, looking up and with looking up and to the right. It is now constant, unilateral and located on the right posterior and lateral aspect of the neck beginning from approximately C4 spinous process and radiates down to around the scapula intermittently but does not radiate past the shoulder or acromioclavicular (AC) joint. In addition, patient complains of intermittent headaches over this same time period that starts over the back of his neck and radiate up over his head, occasionally extending to his forehead with an associated band-like pressure across his temples. There is no associated numbness or tingling in the arms or hands. There is no associated weakness, fine motor deficits, falls or balance problems. He denies symptoms of unintentional weight loss, fevers, incontinence, nausea, vomiting, trouble swallowing, history of malignancy, pain occurring at night or any other symptoms.

He explains he has attempted many different therapies in an attempt to relieve his neck pain including nonsteroidal anti-inflammatory medications, muscle relaxers with modest relief. He briefly tried physiotherapy but quit after a few sessions because he felt it did nothing to improve his pain. In addition

Pain Diagram

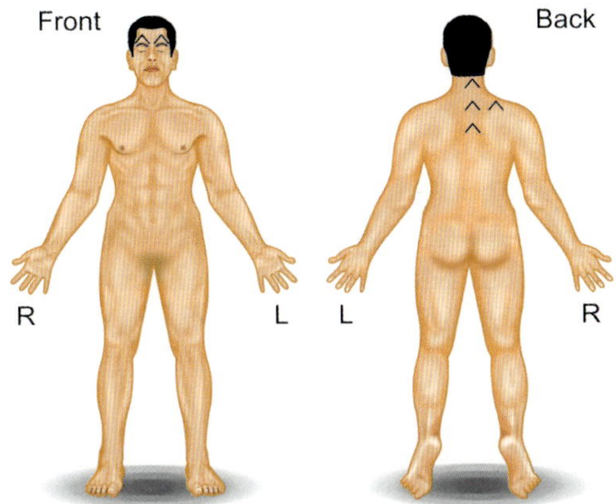

Using the symbols below, the location and type of pain sensations are marked on the diagrams. All the affected areas are included.

TYPE OF SENSATIONS

Aching	∧ ∧ ∧ ∧ ∧ ∧
Sharp or stabbing	X X X X X X
Burning	//////////
Pins and needles	--------------
Numbness	0 0 0 0 0 0

Fig. 10.1: Pain diagram

he has also tried TENS and K-Pads that were prescribed by his primary care physician with moderate relief. He has also sought the advice of a massage therapist and a chiropractor with no relief. He is coming to your office to seek another opinion and to consider the possibility of interventional treatment for his pain.

Patient has aching pain in the right side of the neck and into the trapezius (Fig. 10.1).

PAST MEDICAL HISTORY/PAST SURGICAL HISTORY

Hypertension (HTN), gastroesophageal reflux disease, history of gastric ulcer 5 years previous.

REVIEW OF SYSTEMS

As above, otherwise negative.

FAMILY HISTORY

Mother and father have history of HTN, high-density lipoprotein. No family history of malignancy.

SOCIAL HISTORY

Denies alcohol use other than an occasional glass of wine when out with friends, denies tobacco abuse and denies intravenous or illicit drug use. Employed as an accountant, full time, no workmen's compensation claims.

CURRENT MEDICATIONS

Naprosyn 500 mg BID PRN, cyclobenzaprine 10 mg QHS PRN, hydrochlorothiazide 12.5 mg daily, pantoprazole 40 mg QAM.

ALLERGIES

Penicillin—patient believes he developed hives as a kid.

PHYSICAL EXAMINATION

- *Height*: 6'1"
- *Weight*: 225 lbs
- *Body mass index*: 29.7
- *Pulse*: 76/minute
- *BP*: 129/77 mm Hg
- *Respirations*: 12/minute

He is a pleasant, cooperative man. Looks his stated age, is overweight, and appears in no distress. There are no gait abnormalities and tandem gait is negative for any posterior column or cerebellar signs. Reflexes are 2+ in patellae, Achilles tendons, biceps tendons, pronator teres tendons, and triceps tendons. Babinski is down going, and Hoffman's sign is negative bilaterally. Sensory exam to light touch and pinprick are normal in the upper and lower extremity dermatomes. Manual muscle testing in lower extremities reveals 5/5 strength in bilateral hip flexors, quadriceps, tibialis anterior, extensor halluces longus and gastrocsoleus. Manual muscle testing in upper extremities reveals 5/5 strength in bilateral deltoids, rotator cuff muscles, biceps, extensor carpi radialis, triceps, flexor digitorum profundus and in the intrinsic hand muscles. On shoulder exam, Hawkins test and empty can test are negative bilaterally. There is no AC joint tenderness. Patient has full passive and active range of motions in all four extremities. *There is tenderness to palpation along the right C5-C6 lateral mass. Pain is exacerbated when patient actively and passively rotates neck to the right when cervical spine is in a neutral and extended position. There is palpaple muscle tenderness along cervical paraspinal muscles*. Patient has no pain when active or passive rotation to the left occurs. Spurlings test is negative.

IMAGING

X rays cervical spine AP, lateral, flexion, extension: Normal segmentation, no fracture or spondylolisthesis, *reduced lordosis, mild disc desiccation at C4–5 and C5–6.*

Magnetic resonance imaging cervical spine disc degeneration at C4–5, C5–6.

DIAGNOSIS

Cervical zygapophysial joint (facet) syndrome at C5–C6.

His symptoms are consistent with cervical zygapophysial joint syndrome. While sometimes difficult to diagnose on history and physical exam alone, the syndrome is characterized by axial neck pain that rarely radiates past the shoulder, tends to be unilateral, and an absence of neurological symptoms to suggest myelopathy or radiculopathy.[1-3] In addition the syndrome is also often characterized by pain on passive and active stretch on neck extension and rotation that limits motion.[4]

Other diagnoses in the differential are less likely. Following a motor vehicle accident with significant neck pain, the cervical spine should be cleared of fracture or dislocation via dynamic (flexion and extension) X-rays.[5] The X-rays on this patient were negative, thus pointing to a benign cause for the pain. It is important to always rule out shoulder pathology in patients with a chief complaint of neck pain, and the two may coexist. However, the shoulder exam here is normal and no pain can be elicited. Discogenic neck pain is more likely to have pain on flexion of the neck. With the absence of neurological signs on history or exam, radiculopathy or myelopathy can essentially be ruled out. Due to the length of time and the severity of pain, additional imaging can help confirm this. If an interventional procedure is to be considered, an MRI or CT scan with axial cuts should be obtained prior to injection into the cervical spine.

If the diagnosis remains in doubt, a diagnostic medial branch block can be performed as described below. A block is considered the gold standard for diagnosis.

Treatment Options

An initial recommendation to the patient could be keeping a pain journal as to the time and frequency of neck pain exacerbations. This could help identify activities that make his pain worse and help with lifestyle modifications.

In addition he works as an accountant, and desk jobs are known to promote poor posture which can cause or aggravate neck pain. Good sitting posture should be encouraged. He should also be advised to avoid long periods of sitting and to make efforts to walk around or exercise intermittently during the day. An ergonomic evaluation of his workstation may be ordered. Proper ergonomics may also be emphasized at the time of visit and literature may be provided for patient education.

The importance of physical therapy should be emphasized when treating neck pain and preventing recurrence. Gentle range of motion exercises, light aerobic exercise, and stretching should be advised to the patient. For long-term pain relief, the patient should focus on isometric muscle strengthening which has shown to be beneficial for sources of axial neck pain.[6] In general, the above activities should make patients more involved in their care; however, he has already shown a history of not participating actively in physical therapy.

He already has been taking nonsteroidal anti-inflammatory drugs (NSAIDs) in the form of naprosyn as well as muscle relaxer for pain. A concern for continued NSAID use is his previous history of a gastric ulcer. According to the American College of Gastroenterology patients who are at high risk for gastrointestinal complications, if possible, should consider an alternative to a nonselective NSAID considered such as a selective COX-2 inhibitor used concomitantly with a proton pump inhibitor.[7] Selective COX-2 inhibitors have been shown to have lower risk of gastrointestinal side effects. Evidence for the use of muscle relaxers suggests they are also beneficial, though they are not as strong as they are for NSAIDs.[8]

Other therapeutic alternatives include transcutaneous electrical nerve stimulation, electromagnetic therapy, manual manipulation and massage therapy. However, the evidence that any of these modalities are effective is currently inconclusive.[9-13]

Interventional Options

Cervical zygapophysial joint pain may be addressed in one of three ways: Injection via an intra-articular (Fig. 10.2) approach, injection that "blocks" (anesthesizes) the nerves that supply them (Fig. 10.3), or with radiofrequency neurotomy (Fig. 10.4).

Before each interventional option is discussed it is important to understand the basic anatomy of the cervical zygapophysial joints. Cervical vertebrae C2–C7 have superior and inferior articulating facet joints. The C2–C3 zygapophysial joint is innervated by the dorsal ramus of the third occipital nerve. The remaining cervical zygapophysial joints are innervated by medial branches of the dorsal rami whose roots originate one level rostral and one level caudal to the corresponding joint.[13] For example, the C3–C4 zygapophysial joint is innervated by medial branches of the third and fourth cervical rami, the C4–C5 zygapophysial joint is innervated by medial branches of the fourth and fifth cervical rami, and so on. The following figure illustrates the innervation of the cervical zygapophysial joints. They are taken from Lord et al.[14] and are representation of the variation of the position of the

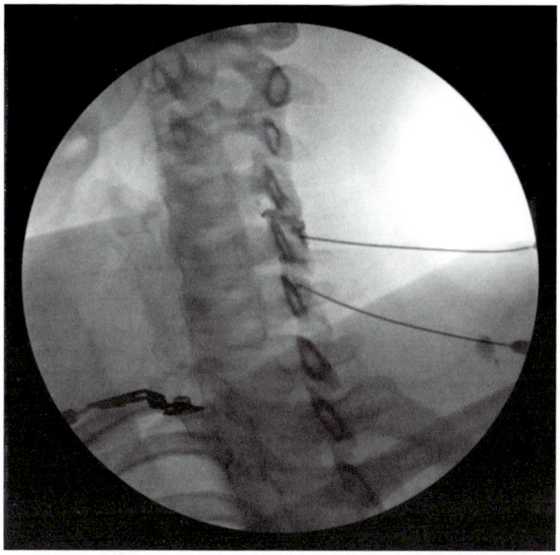

Fig. 10.2: Cervical intra-articular zygapophysial joint injection

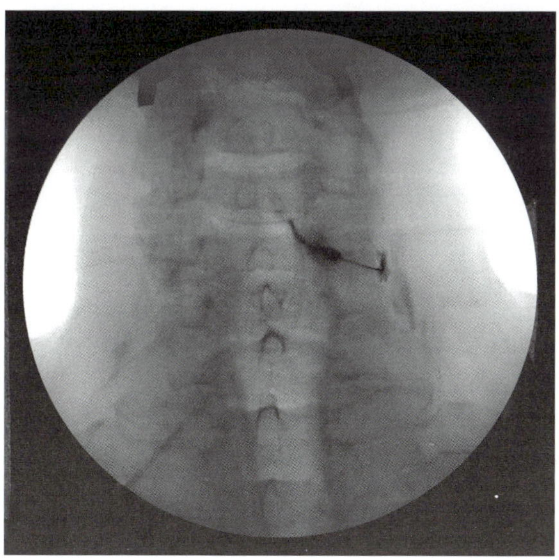

Fig. 10.3: Cervical medial branch block (zygapophysial joint nerve block)

cervical dorsal rami; the lateral view shows the nerves as lines, the antero-posterior view shows them as dots (Fig. 10.5).

Some practitioners advocate trying an intra-articular zygapophysial injection first as steroid can be delivered to the joint itself. If the patient benefits, radiofrequency ablation may be avoided. Unfortunately, studies fail to demonstrate the effectiveness of intra-articular steroid injections.[16] Intra-articular zygapophysial injections are also technically more difficult and may, in cases of significant arthritis, not be possible. There is also a concern

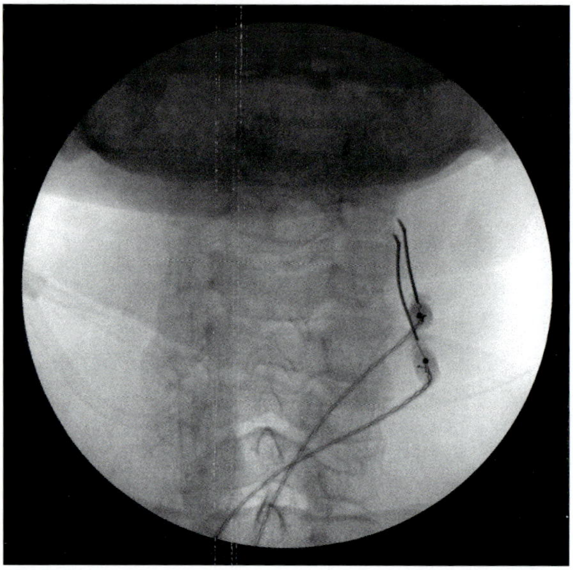

Fig. 10.4: Cervical zygapophysial joint radiofrequency ablation of the third occipital nerve for the right C2-3 zygapophysial joint (anterior posterior view)

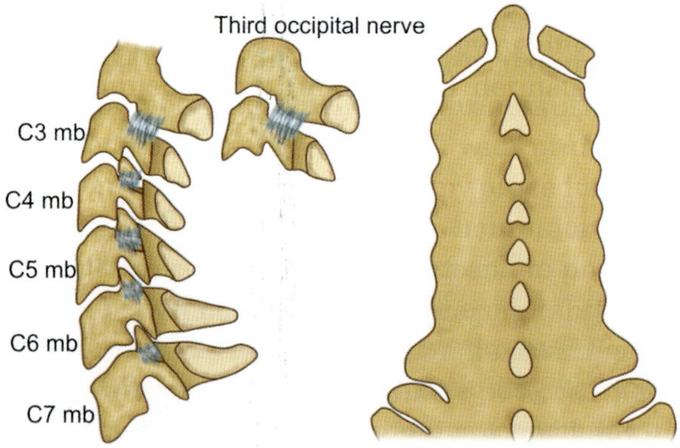

Fig. 10.5: Cervical medial branch anatomy (mb: medial branch nerve)

from a diagnostic standpoint that the anesthetic medicine may extravasate to surrounding tissue and thus reduce the reliability of the diagnostic component.

As recommended by the International Spine Intervention Society (ISIS) and generally accepted as the "gold standard" for diagnosis of facet joint pain, a two positive block paradigm is required for confirming zygapophysial joint pain.[17] The ISIS guidelines say this may include one intra-articular injection and one medial branch block or two medial branch blocks.

Similarly, medial branch block of the dorsal ramus is also predominately used as a diagnostic aid. However, one 2-year trial with follow-up has noted improvement of pain following injection with local anesthetic over a

17–19 weeks period, although the addition of a steroid showed no added benefits of pain relief.[18]

The most studied and most effective interventional technique for short-term relief for cervical zygapophysial joint pain is radiofrequency neurotomy. The landmark study that demonstrated the effectiveness of this procedure demonstrated a mean duration of pain relief defined as a return to 50% of a patient's original pain level of 263 days following radiofrequency neurotomy.[15,19] Since that study was done, there have been several studies to support pain relief from radiofrequency neurotomy in a significant number of patients ranging from months to years.[15,20] Furthermore, evidence suggests that if a patient responds to the first radiofrequency neurotomy well, subsequent procedures will produce a similar satisfaction with pain and a similar duration as the initial injection.[20-22]

Cervical Intra-articular Facet Injection

The patient was prepped and draped sterilely in the prone position with the head rotated to the left after informed consent was signed and all the patient's questions were answered. The risks, benefits, alternative treatment options and prognosis were explained to the patient in the preprocedure area. The risks include, but are not limited to infection, nerve damage, paralysis, allergic reaction, spinal cord injury, epidural hematoma formation, syncope, headache, respiratory or cardiac arrest, death, worse pain and scar formation. All vital signs were monitored prior to, during, and after the procedure. Oxygen saturation was also monitored and noted to be greater than or equal to 94% throughout the procedure. Cardiac monitoring revealed normal sinus rhythm.

The C-arm was positioned so that the region overlying the C5–C6 zygapophysial joint was visualized. The soft tissues overlying these structures were infiltrated with 3–5 cc of 1% lidocaine without epinephrine. A 25-gauge spinal needle was inserted into the superior aspect of the joint. After negative aspirate for blood or CSF, a small volume of nonionic contrast was injected and flow was noted. Radiographs were obtained for documentation purposes. The injectate was administered into the levels noted.

The patient tolerated the procedure well and was discharged after an appropriate period of observation. If there are any complications, the patient was instructed to call us. The patient is to follow-up with the physician as noted above within 2 weeks. The patient was provided with a pain diary noting the preprocedure pain level and asked to bring it to the follow-up appointment.

Cervical Medial Branch Block

The patient was prepped and draped sterilely in the prone position with the head rotated to the left after informed consent was signed and all the patient's questions were answered. The risks, benefits, alternative treatment options and prognosis were explained to the patient in the preprocedure area. The risks include, but are not limited to infection, nerve damage, paralysis, allergic reaction, spinal cord injury, epidural hematoma formation, syncope, headache, respiratory or cardiac arrest, death, worse pain and scar formation. All vital signs were monitored prior to, during, and after the procedure. Oxygen saturation was also monitored and noted to be greater than or equal to 94% throughout the procedure. Cardiac monitoring revealed normal sinus rhythm. The patient was lightly sedated prior to and during the procedure via IV infusion with the anesthesia noted above. The patient remained communicative throughout the procedure.

The C-arm was positioned so that the regions where the C5 and C6 zygapophysial joint nerves are known to reside were visualized. The soft tissues overlying these structures were infiltrated with 3–5 cc of 1% lidocaine without epinephrine for local anesthesia.

For the C3–C7 medial branch nerves, the 25-gauge spinal needle was advanced down to the trough of the lateral masses of each appropriate vertebral level.

An AP projection was used to confirm the positions. After negative aspirate for blood or CSF, a small amount of nonionic contrast was injected and flow of contrast was noted at each level. Radiographs were obtained for documentation purposes. The injectate was administered at the levels noted above.

The patient tolerated the procedure well and was discharged after an appropriate period of observation. If there are any complications, the patient was instructed to call us. The patient is to follow-up with the physician as noted above within 1–2 weeks.

The patient was also given a pain diary and was instructed to note the pain level and activities at the time of entering the data for the day of the procedure. The patient will bring this data to the follow-up appointment for diagnostic purposes.

Cervical Medial Branch Radiofrequency Ablation

The patient was prepped and draped sterilely in the prone position with the head rotated to the left after informed consent was signed and all the patient's questions were answered. The risks, benefits, alternative treatment options and prognosis were explained to the patient in the preprocedure area. The risks include, but are not limited to infection, nerve damage, paralysis, allergic reaction, spinal cord injury, epidural hematoma formation, syncope, headache, respiratory or cardiac arrest, death, worse pain and scar formation. All vital signs were monitored prior to, during, and after the procedure. Oxygen saturation was also monitored and noted to be greater than or equal to 94% throughout the procedure. Cardiac monitoring revealed

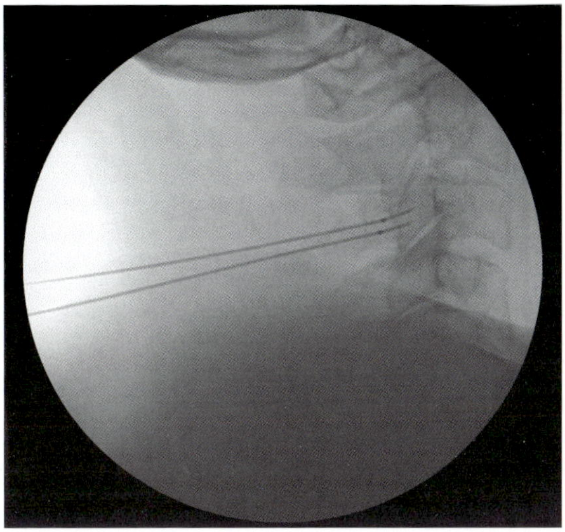

Fig. 10.6: Cervical zygapophysial joint radiofrequency ablation of the third occipital nerve for the right C2-C3 zygapophysial joint (lateral view)

normal sinus rhythm. The patient was lightly sedated prior to and during the procedure via IV infusion with the anesthesia noted above. The patient remained communicative throughout the procedure. A grounding pad was placed on the patient.

The C-arm was positioned so that the appropriate vertebral levels for the above mentioned zygapophysial joint nerves were visualized. The soft tissues overlying these structures were infiltrated with 2–6 cc of 1% lidocaine without epinephrine.

At the C5 and C6 medial branch nerves, the radiofrequency needle was advanced down to the trough of the lateral masses of each vertebral level. A lateral projection was used to confirm the positions. At both levels, the radiofrequency needle stylets were replaced with the radiofrequency probes. Impedance was noted to be less than 300 Ω at both levels. Sensory stimulation at 50 Hz and motor stimulation at 2 Hz were performed at each level to ensure no radicular stimulation and to observe maximal multifidus contractions. An additional 1–2 cc of 1% lidocaine without epinephrine was infiltrated into the soft tissues. Subsequently at each level, lesioning was performed at 80°C for approximately 90 seconds. The lesioning was repeated two times at each level for 90 seconds. At the cessation of the procedure, a small mixture of betamethasone and 1% lidocaine without epinephrine was injected and the needles removed. Radiographs were obtained for documentation purposes.

The patient tolerated the procedure well, was taken to the recovery room and then discharged after an appropriate period of observation. If there are any complications, the patient was instructed to call us. The patient is to follow-up with the physician as noted above within 2–3 weeks (Fig. 10.6).

REFERENCES

1. Dwyer A, Aprill C, Bogduk N. Cervical zygapophyseal joint pain patterns. I: A study in normal volunteers. Spine (Phila Pa 1976). 1990;15(6): 453-7.
2. Cooper G, Bailey B, Bogduk N. Cervical zygapophysial joint pain maps. Pain Med. 2007;8(4):344-53.
3. Aprill C, Dwyer A, Bogduk N. Cervical zygapophyseal joint pain patterns. II: A clinical evaluation. Spine (Phila Pa 1976). 1990;15(6):458-61.
4. van Eerd M, Patijn J, Lataster A, et al. 5. Cervical facet pain. Pain Pract. 2010;10(2):113-23.
5. Clancy MJ. Clearing the cervical spine of adult victims of trauma. J Accid Emerg Med. 1999; 16(3):208-14.
6. Ylinen J, Takala EP, Nykanen M, et al. Active neck muscle training in the treatment of chronic neck pain in women: a randomized controlled trial. JAMA. 2003;289(19):2509-16.
7. Lanza FL, Chan FK, Quigley EM, et al. Guidelines for prevention of NSAID-related ulcer complications. Am J Gastroenterol. 2009;104(3):728-38.
8. Deyo RA. Drug therapy for back pain. Which drugs help which patients? Spine (Phila Pa 1976). 1996;21(24):2840-9; discussion 2849-50.
9. Kroeling P, Gross A, Houghton PE, et al. Electrotherapy for neck disorders. Cochrane Database Syst Rev. 2005;(2):CD004251.
10. Patel KC, Gross A, Graham N, et al. Massage for mechanical neck disorders. Cochrane Database Syst Rev. 2012;9:CD004871.
11. Gross AR, Hoving JL, Haines TA, et al. A Cochrane review of manipulation and mobilization for mechanical neck disorders. Spine (Phila Pa 1976). 2004;29 (1-4):1541-8.
12. Hurwitz EL, Carragee EJ, van der Velde G, et al. Treatment of neck pain: noninvasive interventions: results of the Bone and Joint Decade 2000-2010 Task Force on Neck Pain and Its Associated Disorders. Spine (Phila Pa 1976). 2008; 33(4 Suppl):S123-52.
13. Bogduk N. The clinical anatomy of the cervical dorsal rami. Spine. 1982;7(4): 319-30.
14. Lord SM, Barnsley L, Bogduk N. Percutaneous radiofrequency neurotomy in the treatment of cervical zygapophysial joint pain: a caution. Neurosurgery. 1995;36(4):732-9.
15. Lord SM, Barnsley L, Wallis BJ, et al. Percutaneous radio-frequency neurotomy for chronic cervical zygapophyseal-joint pain. N Engl J Med. 1996;335(23): 1721-6.
16. Falco FJ, Erhart S, Wargo BW, et al. Systematic review of diagnostic utility and therapeutic effectiveness of cervical facet joint interventions. Pain Physician. 2009;12(2):323-44.
17. Bogduk N. Spinal Diagnostic and Treatment Procedures: Practice Guidelines, 1st edition. San Francisco, CA: International Spine Intervention Society; 2004.
18. Manchikanti L, Singh V, Falco FJ, et al. Cervical medial branch blocks for chronic cervical facet joint pain: a randomized, double-blind, controlled trial with one-year follow-up. Spine (Phila Pa 1976). 2008;33(17):1813-20.
19. Niemisto L, Kalso E, Malmivaara A, et al. Radiofrequency denervation for neck and back pain. A systematic review of randomized controlled trials. Cochrane Database Syst Rev. 2003;(1):CD004058.

20. Falco FJ, Manchikanti L, Datta S, et al. Systematic review of the therapeutic effectiveness of cervical facet joint interventions: an update. Pain Physician. 2012;15(6):E839-68.
21. Barnsley L. Percutaneous radiofrequency neurotomy for chronic neck pain: outcomes in a series of consecutive patients. Pain Med. 2005;6(4):282-6.
22. MacVicar J, Borowczyk JM, MacVicar AM, et al. Cervical medial branch radiofrequency neurotomy in New Zealand. Pain Med. 2012;13(5):647-54.

11

Hip Pain

Anupam Sinha, Madhuri Dholakia

CHIEF COMPLAINT

The patient complains of left hip pain.

HISTORY OF PRESENT ILLNESS

A 66-year-old male with no past significant medical history presents with a 3 month history of insidious left groin and thigh pain. He denies any trauma or injury. He denies any low back pain but does report some left buttock discomfort. It is aching at rest, sharp with standing and walking. His pain is worse with weight bearing on the left leg, walking, and getting in and out of his car. He reports five out of ten pain radiating from the left groin into the medial thigh. He denies any lower extremity weakness or paresthesia. He denies any bowel, bladder or balance disturbance. There is no unintentional weight loss, fevers, chills or night sweats.

Treatments to date have included over the counter medications, heat and ice packs, and a trigger point injection into the greater trochanteric region from his primary physician; he has had no relief with these options.

Note the aching pain in the left groin and buttocks (Fig. 11.1).

PAST MEDICAL HISTORY/PAST SURGICAL HISTORY

None

REVIEW OF SYSTEMS

Otherwise negative

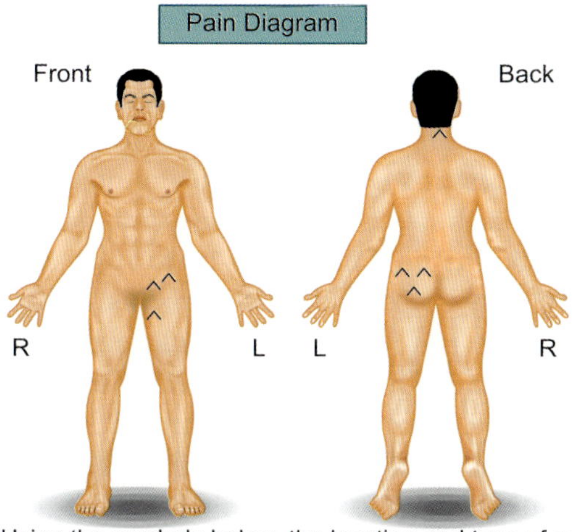

Using the symbols below, the location and type of pain sensations are marked on the diagrams. All the affected areas are included.

TYPE OF SENSATIONS

Aching	^ ^ ^ ^ ^ ^
Sharp or stabbing	X X X X X X
Burning	//////////
Pins and needles	--------------
Numbness	0 0 0 0 0 0

Fig. 11.1: Pain diagram. Note the aching pain in the left groin and buttocks

FAMILY HISTORY

Parents alive with no medical issues

SOCIAL HISTORY

Does not drink or smoke, married, retired, avid golfer.

CURRENT MEDICATIONS

Ibuprofen 600 mg BID PRN

ALLERGIES

None

PHYSICAL EXAMINATION

- *Height*: 5'11"
- *Weight*: 200 lbs

- *Pulse*: 75/minute
- *BP*: 120/80 mm Hg
- *Respirations*: 16/minute

General Appearance

Pleasant, cooperative, looks stated age, in no distress.

Gait and tandem gait stable. Able to heel walk and toe walk without difficulty. Pulses are 2+ in the radial and dorsalis pedis arteries. Babinski testing reveals downgoing toes bilaterally. Slump test and supine straight leg raise to 90° are negative bilaterally. No tenderness over the lumbar spinous processes. *Patrick's test is positive on the left. Internal rotation of the left hip reproduces groin and thigh pain. Stinchfield's test is positive on the left.* No tenderness to palpation over the bilateral trochanteric bursae. No tenderness over the sacroiliac joints. Manual muscle testing in the lower limbs reveals 5/5 bilateral hip flexors, quadriceps, tibialis anterior, extensor hallucis longus, and gastroc soleus; however, there is trace weakness in the left hip flexor due to pain. Sensory examination to light touch and pinprick is normal in the lower extremity dermatomes. Proprioception is intact at the great toes bilaterally. Normal muscle tone. Reflexes are 2+ in patellae, medial hamstrings and Achilles tendons. No ankle clonus bilaterally.

IMAGING

X-rays of the pelvis reveal moderate degenerative joint disease in the left hip without evidence of fracture.

DIAGNOSIS

Left Hip Degenerative Joint Disease

Osteoarthritis of the hip is one of the most common causes of gait dysfunction among older adults in the United States (knee osteoarthritis being the other).[1] Risk factors that may increase the likelihood of developing hip osteoarthritis include: genetic predisposition, childhood developmental hip dysplasia, avascular necrosis, femoral acetabular impingement, prior hip trauma or fracture, and obesity.[1] Early symptoms of hip osteoarthritis may include: groin, buttock, and/or thigh pain, pain with weight bearing, hip joint stiffness, and referred knee pain. As the arthritis becomes more severe, the patient may develop an antalgic gait pattern, joint deformity, hip girdle weakness, and leg length discrepancy.[2] The classic radiographic features of osteoarthritis of the hip are joint space narrowing, osteophyte formation, subchondral cyst formation and subchondral sclerosis.[2]

Treatment Options

Physical therapy and exercise for strengthening of the hip girdle muscles may improve overall hip joint stability and increase flexibility.[3] Heat and cold modalities may also help reduce hip joint pain and inflammation.[4] Anti-inflammatories (nonsteroidal anti-inflammatory drugs) and acetaminophen may be used to reduce symptoms of arthritic joint pain.[4] While helpful in knee osteoarthritis, glucosamine chondroitin has been found to have no impact on pain, disease progression, or functional status for hip osteoarthritis.[5] Ultimately, total hip arthroplasty (THA) may provide the most relief in patients with moderate to severe osteoarthritis.[6]

Image-guided intra-articular injections of steroid and anesthetic may also alleviate discomfort from mild to moderate hip osteoarthritis.[7] These injections may be done under fluoroscopy or musculoskeletal ultrasound. Care must be taken when injecting to avoid the femoral vessels (nerve, artery and vein) which course along the proximal anterior thigh. There is limited data on how frequently it is safe to administer steroid injections to patients with hip osteoarthritis. Repeat injections more than four times annually are generally not recommended.[7] Previous studies have suggested avoiding the use of intra-articular steroids injected in the hip for at least 2 months before total hip arthroplasty due to an increased risk of postoperative infection.[8,9] A more recent study suggests an intra-articular steroid injection through a lateral approach to the hip is safe when performed using strictly aseptic technique. However, caution is still advised when planning a THA within 2 months after an intra-articular steroid injection (Fig. 11.2).[10]

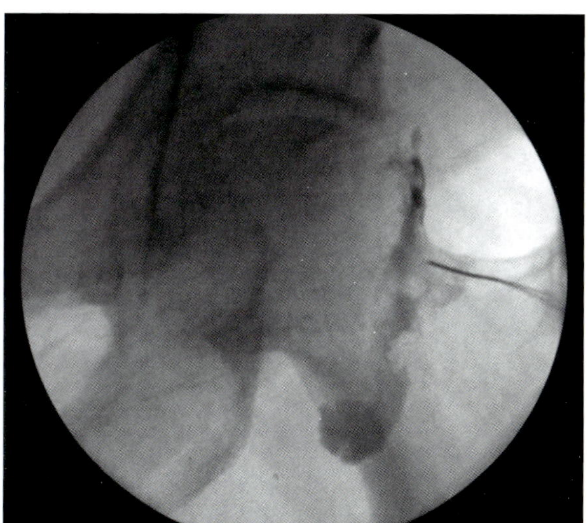

Fig. 11.2: Intra-articular hip injection. Note the flow of contrast into the capsule and the characteristic "ring sign" of contrast in the joint

The patient was prepped and draped in a sterile fashion in the supine position after informed consent was signed and all the patient's questions were answered, including the risks, benefits, alternative treatment options and prognosis. The risks include but are not limited to infection, allergic reaction, nerve damage, paralysis, syncope, and worsening pain. All vital signs were monitored prior to, during, and after the procedure. Oxygen saturation was also monitored and noted to be greater than or equal to 94% throughout the procedure. Cardiac monitoring revealed normal sinus rhythm.

The C-arm was positioned so that the region overlying the femoral acetabular junction was visualized. The femoral pulse was palpated. Staying lateral to the pulse, the soft tissues overlying the joint were infiltrated with 3–5 cc of 1% lidocaine without epinephrine. A 22-gauge spinal needle was inserted and directed toward the femoral neck until bony contact. After negative aspirate for blood, a total volume of 3.5 cc of nonionic contrast was injected and flow of contrast was noted. Radiographs were obtained for documentation purposes. The injectate was administered.

The patient tolerated the procedure well and was discharged after an appropriate period of observation. If there are any complications, the patient was instructed to call us. The patient is to follow-up with the physician as noted above within 2–3 weeks.

REFERENCES

1. Suri P, Morgenroth DC, Hunter DJ. Epidemiology of osteoarthritis and associated comorbidities. PM R. 2012;4(5 Suppl):S10-9.
2. JF Sarwark (Ed). Essentials of Musculoskeletal Care, fourth edition. Rosemont, IL, American Academy of Orthopaedic Surgeons; 2010.
3. Fransen M, McConnell S, Hernandez-Molina G, et al. Does land-based exercise reduce pain and disability associated with hip osteoarthritis? A meta-analysis of randomized controlled trials. Osteoarthritis Cartilage. 2010;18(5):613-20.
4. Hochberg MC, Altman RD, April KT, et al. American College of Rheumatology 2012 recommendations for the use of nonpharma-cologic and pharmacologic therapies in osteoarthritis of the hand, hip, and knee. Arthritis Care Res (Hoboken). 2012;64(4):465-74.
5. Reichenbach S, Sterchi R, Scherer M, et al. Meta-analysis: chondroitin for osteoarthritis of the knee or hip. AnnIntern Med. 2007;146(8):580-90.
6. Grayson CW, Decker RC. Total joint arthroplasty for persons with osteoarthritis. PM R. 2012;4(5 Suppl):S97-103.
7. Zhang W, Moskowitz RW, Nuki G, et al. OARSI recommendations for the management of hip and knee osteoarthritis, Part II: OARSI evidence-based, expert consensus guidelines. Osteoarthritis Cartilage. 2008;16(2):137-62.
8. McIntosh AL, Hanssen AD, Wenger DE, et al. Recent intraarticular steroid injection may increase infection rates in primary THA. Clin Orthop Relat Res. 2006;451:50-4.
9. Kaspar S, de V de Beer J. Infection in hip arthroplasty after previous injection of steroid. J Bone Joint Surg Br. 2005;87(4):454-7.
10. Meermans G, Corten K, Simon JP. Is the infection rate in primary THA increased after steroid injection? Clin Orthop Relat Res. 2012;470(11):3213-9.

12 Complex Regional Pain Syndrome—Lower Extremity

Jeremy Simon, Matthew McAuliffe

CHIEF COMPLAINT

The patient complains of pain and cold feeling in the left foot (Fig. 12.1).

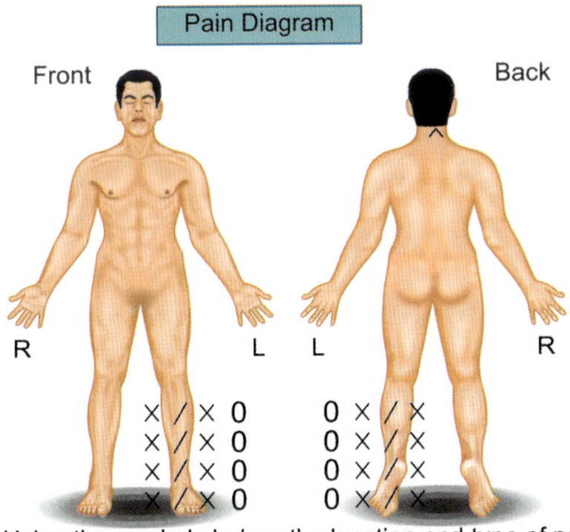

Using the symbols below, the location and type of pain sensations are marked on the diagrams. All the affected areas are included.

TYPE OF SENSATIONS

Aching	^ ^ ^ ^ ^ ^
Sharp or stabbing	X X X X X X
Burning	//////////
Pins and needles	--------------
Numbness	0 0 0 0 0 0

Fig. 12.1: Pain diagram

HISTORY OF PRESENT ILLNESS

This patient is a very pleasant, 10-year-old right-handed female who injured her left foot 2 months ago. She twisted her left foot and ankle while playing volleyball. She was placed in an air cast and diagnosed with a bone contusion by a local sports medicine doctor. When she was at school, another student "stepped on it" and then she developed the above pain syndrome. The pain has been constant and severe. It is associated with a cold feeling in the entire left foot. It has been also been changing colors and is "blue/purplish looking". She never had symptoms like this prior to these incidents. She went to an orthopedic surgeon who had performed X-rays as well as an MRI of the left foot and a whole-body bone scan. The X-rays were negative for fracture. The MRI demonstrated bone contusions and edema without fracture or ligamentous injury. The bone scan was consistent with complex regional pain syndrome (CRPS). The symptoms have not gotten any better. She rates her pain about 7/10 and it is constant. It is aggravated with walking. Light touch increases pain and even sheets touching the foot or wearing socks aggravate it. It is described as burning and cold in quality. She is presently using crutches to walk. There are no similar symptoms on the right side. There is no back pain and no radiating pain from the proximal limb. She denies weakness. She denies any bowel or bladder incontinence, unintentional weight loss or weight gain, fevers, chills, or night sweats. She denies any history of cancer, tuberculosis, infections, autoimmune disorders or other significant medical problems.

TREATMENTS TO DATE

Ibuprofen 200 mg TID PRN, crutches, attempted physical therapy, but discontinued due to severe pain after one attempt.

PAST MEDICAL HISTORY

None; normal development, normal intelligence

PAST SURGICAL HISTORY

None

REVIEW OF SYSTEMS

Positive for pain and temperature changes in the right foot

FAMILY HISTORY

Significant for blood clots in her father. Both her parents are alive. Her mother accompanies her today.

SOCIAL HISTORY

She denies tobacco, alcohol, or illegal drugs. She is a fourth grade student at a local elementary school; Lives with both of her parents. She is an only child.

CURRENT MEDICATIONS

Ibuprofen 200 mg TID PRN

ALLERGIES

Penicillin

PHYSICAL EXAMINATION

- *Height*: 4'1"
- *Weight*: 80 pounds
- *Blood pressure*: 108/60 mm Hg
- *Pulse*: 88/minute
- *Respirations*: 16/minute

Gait and tandem gait stable. Romberg sign is negative. *She has an antaegic gait with the inability to bear weight on the left foot.* Pulses are 2+ in the radial and dorsalis pedis arteries. Babinski testing reveals downgoing toes bilaterally. Slump test and supine straight leg raised to 90° are negative bilaterally; Negative femoral nerve stretch test bilaterally. No palpable step-off in the lumbar spine. No pain with extension or rotation. No tenderness over the lumbar spinous processes. No palpable scoliotic curve. No lumbar segmental tenderness. No palpable muscle spasm in the lumbar paraspinals. Patrick's test is negative bilaterally. Internal rotation of the hips does not cause pain. No tenderness to palpation over the bilateral trochanteric bursae. Negative Gaenslen's sign, negative Thomas test, negative Ober's test bilaterally. No tenderness over the sacroiliac joints. Manual muscle testing in the lower limbs reveals 5/5 bilateral hip flexors, quadriceps, tibialis anterior, extensor hallucis longus and gastroc soleus. *There is pain limited strength in the left tibialis anterior, extensor hallicus longus and flexor hallicus longus. Decreased sensation to light touch and allodynia in the dorsal, lateral, plantar and medial aspects of her foot on the left side. Active range of motion in the left ankle is markedly reduced in all directions; passive range of motion is exquisitely painful.* Proprioception is intact at the great toes bilaterally. Normal muscle tone. Reflexes are 2+ in patellae, medial hamstrings and Achilles tendons. No ankle clonus bilaterally.

She has a mottled appearing foot with dystrophic changes in the entire left foot.

IMAGING

X-rays left foot: negative for fracture, dislocation.

Whole body bone scan: demonstrates markedly reduced flow and uptake in the left foot.

Magnetic resonance imaging left foot: Marrow edema of the medial sesamoid bone at the first metatarsophalangeal joint due to contusion/stress response. Diffuse subcutaneous edema.

DIAGNOSIS

Complex regional pain syndrome Type I: Left foot.

Complex Regional Pain Syndrome

The first descriptions of sympathetically mediated pain (SMP) were from Claude Bernard in the mid 1800s.[1] Silas Weir-Mitchell first described "causalgia" in American Civil War veterans. Formerly known as reflex sympathetic dystrophy (RSD) and causalgia, in 1994, the International Association for the Study of Pain (IASP) changed the names of these entities to CRPS, Types I and II. They are treated as the same condition, but Type II is distinguished by a documented injury to a nerve.[1]

The clinical characteristics of CRPS Type I typically occurs secondary to a crush injury, tight fitting casts, soft tissue injury and immobilization. CRPS Type II occurs with a documented nerve injury such as a penetrating injury or iatrogenic disruption, as in a surgical procedure. A series of symptoms then develop including pain that is much more severe than to be expected from the event, avoidance of weight-bearing or use of the extremity, allodynia/hyperesthesia of the affected area, temperature changes, swelling, skin color changes and/or sudomotor changes.[2]

The pathophysiology of CRPS types I and II remain elusive and are not completely understood. Current research suggests that both central and peripheral sensitization of nerves occurs.[3] The mechanism may involve chronic activation of the afferent C-fibers from a noxious stimulus and subsequent reduction in the threshold for activation.[4]

Evidence supporting the central sensitization theory of CRPS includes a study which showed reorganization of cortical somatosensory representation as demonstrated by magnetoencephalography.[5] Furthermore, it was found that the cortical reorganization was reversible with resolution of symptoms in patients with CRPS.[6,7]

N-methyl D-aspartate (NMDA) receptors are believed to play a pivotal role in central sensitization via plasticity of neural substrates.[8] When afferent nerves are more sensitive to neurotransmitter release, action potentials are produced at lower levels of stimulation.[8] This makes nerves more "sensitive" to neurotransmitter release and as a result nociceptive transmission is enhanced through increased NMDA receptor activation.[8]

It is thought that peripheral sensitization may be related to chronic neurogenic inflammation. Often patients will complain of signs of inflammation including erythema or skin color changes and pain. Evidence that supports this theory includes a study showing higher skin blister fluid levels of IL-6 and TNF-α found in CRPS patients on the side of the affected limb.[9] Another study supporting neurogenic inflammation showed increased serum levels of substance P in patients with CRPS.[10]

As the earlier term RSD implied, the sympathetic nervous system is still believed to play a role in the condition. Some advocated a subcategory for CRPS involving sympathetic hyperactivity as SMP. This subset of CRPS is diagnosed after a positive response to sympathetic blockade.[11] This subset refers to the presumed mechanism of continued pain, not the clinical picture.[12]

The early autonomic-type symptoms may be the result of effects on the ability of the vessels to constrict or dilate.[13] The symptoms early on may be warmth in the affected body part, but later coolness often develops. In addition, other symptoms of autonomic dysfunction are frequently present in CRPS such as hyperhidrosis and differences in skin blood flow in the affected body part.[14]

The diagnosis of CRPS is largely clinical. Criteria exist as described by the IASP in 1994.[3,12] For CRPS Type I, this includes:

- Presence of noxious event/immobilization
- Ongoing pain, allodynia/hyperesthesia out of proportion to event
- Evidence at some time of edema, vascular changes (reduced or increased skin temperature), or abnormal sudomotor changes
- Exclusion of other explanations

Budapest criteria as taken from Harden RN, Bruehl S, Stanton-Hicks M, et al. for making a diagnosis of CRPS type I:[15]

To make the clinical diagnosis, the following criteria must be met:

- Continuing pain, which is disproportionate to any inciting event
- Must report at least one symptom in three of the four following categories:
  - *Sensory: Reports of hyperesthesia and/or allodynia*
  - *Vasomotor: Reports of temperature asymmetry and/or skin color changes and/or skin color asymmetry*
  - *Sudomotor/edema: Reports of edema and/or sweating changes and/or sweating asymmetry*

  - *Motor/trophic: Reports of decreased range of motion and/or motor dysfunction (weakness, tremor, dystonia) and/or trophic changes (hair, nail, skin)*
- Must display at least one sign at time of evaluation in two or more of the following categories:
  - *Sensory: Evidence of hyperalgesia (to pinprick) and/or allodynia (to light touch and/or temperature sensation and/or deep somatic pressure and/or joint movement)*
  - *Vasomotor: Evidence of temperature asymmetry (> 1°C) and/or skin color changes and/or asymmetry*
  - *Sudomotor/edema: Evidence of edema and/or sweating changes and/or sweating asymmetry*
  - *Motor/trophic: Evidence of decreased range of motion and/or motor dysfunction (weakness, tremor, dystonia) and/or trophic changes (hair, nail, skin)*
- There is no other diagnosis that better explains the signs and symptoms

For Type II, the criteria are the same, but a documented nerve injury has occurred.

A triple-phase bone scan may show homogeneous hypoperfusion in the perfusion and blood-pool phases. There may also be increased periarticular uptake in the delayed images.

TREATMENT OPTIONS

There is no single cure for CRPS and it is often managed with multiple approaches. Typically, a combination of physical therapy and medications in different classes are prescribed. Sympathetic nerve blocks and rarely surgery or chemical sympathectomy may be employed. The ultimate goal is to improve a patient's functional status.

Although there is no single cure for CRPS, there is evidence that in some cases it can be prevented. One study demonstrated early mobilization and physical therapy significantly decreased the incidence of CRPS in patients with hemiplegia.[16] Therefore it is important to begin early physical therapy in patients who have limbs that may be at risk of developing CRPS.

Physical therapy with desensitization and forced weight bearing is an essential element in the treatment of CRPS. The primary goal is to improve the function of the affected part. Altering modalities are utilized to desensitize the painful area. This may involve exposing the skin to soft or silken to gradually rougher materials. Varying degrees of pressure are also employed. The goal is to diminish, and hopefully extinguish, allodynia and hyperesthesia. There is mixed evidence supporting the benefits of physical therapy in CRPS, and the evidence suggests as the symptoms of CRPS progress, physical therapy is less likely to benefit.[17,18] However, it should be stressed, that the risks of

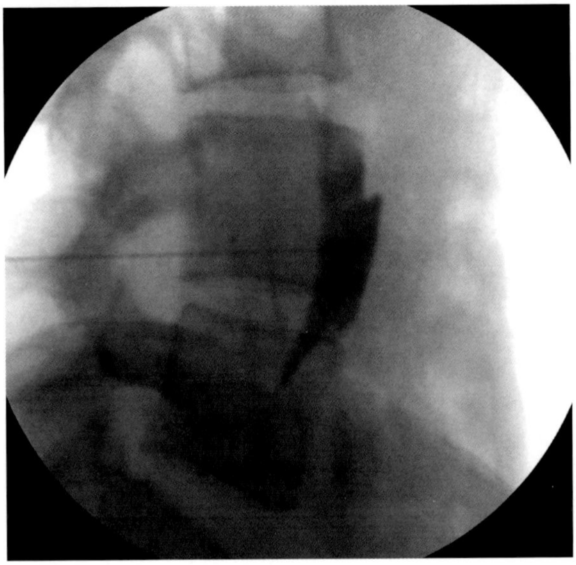

Fig. 12.2: Lateral view confirming contrast placement along the region of the sympathetic chain without vascular flow

implementing a physical therapy program in patients is low, and should be a first line consideration in treatment of CRPS.

Medications are often used in a variety of classes with limited data on their true benefit in CRPS.[19] Oral steroids may be considered early in the diagnosis.[20] Nonsteroidal anti-inflammatory medications may also provide some analgesic benefit. Neuropathic pain medications such as the tricyclic antidepressants (e.g. amitriptyline, nortriptyline) may be considered and the mechanisms of action are described elsewhere in this book. Bisphosphonate medications are often used in CRPS.[21] The mechanism of action is to reduce bone turnover, which is often overactive in this condition.[22]

The practice of infusing ketamine under monitored conditions is under investigation.[23] Intravenous ketamine is believed to inhibit the sympathetic-mediated pain via ketamine's blockade of NMDA-receptors.[24] This treatment has been utilized in the outpatient as well as inpatient setting and is employed in refractory cases.[25,26]

Blockade of the sympathetic chain via the injection of bupivacaine may be considered, especially early in the acute phase of CRPS (Fig. 12.2). This procedure is normally performed under fluoroscopic guidance for safety and specificity. The temperature of the affected extremity is monitored, often with a transdermal thermometer. After the injection of anesthetic, a positive response will result in vasodilation and thus a significant increase in temperature in the treated limb. The patient should also exhibit a significant decrease in their pain.

If a lumbar sympathetic block is performed, it is ideally followed immediately or within 30 minutes by a physical therapy program. As previously mentioned, the goals are to promote weight-bearing and desensitization of the affected limb while the sympathetic nerve fibers are anesthetized.

Positive results with sympathetic block are directly correlated with symptom duration, younger age. A recent study suggests that allodynia and hypoesthesia were negative predictors for a good result with sympathetic block and that no factors were indicative of who would respond to this injection.[27]

Risks associated with lumbar sympathetic blockade include bleeding into the retroperitoneum and psoas muscles, puncture of the inferior vena cava or aorta, infection/abscess formation, kidney or ureteral puncture, direct neural injury, seizure, arrhythmia, syncope, death and paralysis. Patients with a bleeding diathesis or who are on blood thinning medications require particular attention as they may be at increased risk for severe bleeding complications. Vital signs should be monitored prior to, during and after the procedure.

Other invasive strategies are in use for CRPS. Some advocate a sympathectomy for refractory cases. This may be accomplished surgically via open resection of the lumbar sympathetic chain on the affected side, chemically via injection of alcohol or phenol, or with percutaneous radiofrequency ablation.[27,28] Results of these treatments are variable and are typically considered in very refractory and debilitating cases of CRPS with SMP.[5,29,30]

PLAN

Due to the duration of symptoms, the classic signs and symptoms of CRPS, the significant debility, and lack of tolerance to a therapy program and other conservative treatments, it was mutually decided with the patient and her family to go forward with a left L3 sympathetic block under fluoroscopy. Arrangements were made in advance to the procedure with the in-house physical therapists to begin an immediate desensitization and forced weight-bearing program following the injection.

SAMPLE DICTATION

A skin thermometer was placed on the affected limb prior to the procedure and informed consent was signed. All the patient's questions were answered, including the risks, benefits, alternative treatment options and prognosis. The risks include but are not limited to infection, retroperitoneal bleed, kidney or ureteral puncture, nerve damage, paralysis, epidural hematoma, syncope, headache, allergic reaction, cardiac arrest, and scar formation. The patient was placed in the prone position and the target area was sterilely prepped. Vital signs and oxygen saturation were monitored pre and periprocedurally. Cardiac monitoring revealed normal sinus rhythm.

The C-arm was positioned so that an oblique view of the region overlying the inferior portion of the L2 or L3 vertebral body was visualized. The soft tissues overlying this structure were anesthetized with an injection of 1% lidocaine without epinephrine. A 22-gauge spinal needle was inserted down to the inferior anterolateral aspect of the L2 or L3 vertebral body. After negative aspirate for blood or CSF, a 2-4 cc volume of contrast dye was injected into the region where the sympathetic chain is known to reside and flow of contrast was noted, ensuring nonvascular and proper spread. Radiographs were obtained for documentation purposes. An injectate consisting of 10 cc of 0.25% bupivacaine was slowly injected. The needle was then removed and an occlusive dressing was placed on the insertion site.

The patient tolerated the procedure well and was discharged after an appropriate period of observation. If there are any complications, the patient was instructed to call us. The patient is to follow-up with the physician as noted above within 2–3 weeks.

REFERENCES

1. Harden RN, Oaklander AL, Burton AW, et al. Complex regional pain syndrome: practical diagnostic and treatment guidelines, 4th edition. Pain Med. 2013;14(2):180-229.
2. Field J. Complex Regional Pain Syndrome: a review. J Hand Surg Eur Vol. 2013;38(6):616-26.
3. Marinus J, Moseley GL, Birklein F, et al. Clinical features and pathophysiology of complex regional pain syndrome. Lancet Neurol. 2011;10(7):637-48.
4. Pappagallo M, Rosenberg AD. Epidemiology, pathophysiology, and management of complex regional pain syndrome. Pain Pract. 2001;1(1):11-20.
5. Straube S, Derry S, Moore RA, et al. Cervico-thoracic or lumbar sympathectomy for neuropathic pain and complex regional pain syndrome. Cochrane Database Syst Rev. 2010;(7):CD002918.
6. Maihofner C, Handwerker HO, Neundorfer B, et al. Cortical reorganization during recovery from complex regional pain syndrome. Neurology. 2004;63(4):693-701.
7. Pleger B, Tegenthoff M, Ragert P, et al. Sensorimotor retuning [corrected] in complex regional pain syndrome parallels pain reduction. Ann Neurol. 2005;57(3):425-9.
8. Zhou HY, Chen SR, Pan HL. Targeting N-methyl-D-aspartate receptors for treatment of neuropathic pain. Expert Rev Clin Pharmacol. 2011;4(3):379-88.
9. Wesseldijk F, Huygen FJ, Heijmans-Antonissen C, et al. Six years follow-up of the levels of TNF-alpha and IL-6 in patients with complex regional pain syndrome type 1. Mediators Inflamm. 2008;2008:469439.
10. Leis S, Weber M, Isselmann A, et al. Substance-P-induced protein extravasation is bilaterally increased in complex regional pain syndrome. Exp Neurol. 2003; 183(1):197-204.
11. Stanton-Hicks M, Janig W, Hassenbusch S, et al. Reflex sympathetic dystrophy: changing concepts and taxonomy. Pain. 1995;63(1):127-33.
12. Loeser. Bonica's Management of Pain; 2001.

13. Wasner G, Schattschneider J, Heckmann K, et al. Vascular abnormalities in reflex sympathetic dystrophy (CRPS I): mechanisms and diagnostic value. Brain. 2001;124(Pt 3):587-99.
14. Wasner G. Vasomotor disturbances in complex regional pain syndrome--a review. Pain Med. 2010;11(8):1267-73.
15. Harden RN, Bruehl S, Stanton-Hicks M, et al. Proposed new diagnostic criteria for complex regional pain syndrome. Pain Med. 2007;8(4):326-31.
16. Braus DF, Krauss JK, Strobel J. The shoulder-hand syndrome after stroke: a prospective clinical trial. Ann Neurol. 1994;36(5):728-33.
17. Oerlemans HM, Goris JA, de Boo T, et al. Do physical therapy and occupational therapy reduce the impairment percentage in reflex sympathetic dystrophy? American journal of physical medicine & rehabilitation / Assoc Acad Physiatrists. 1999;78:533-9.
18. Oerlemans HM, Oostendorp RA, de Boo T, et al. Pain and reduced mobility in complex regional pain syndrome I: outcome of a prospective randomised controlled clinical trial of adjuvant physical therapy versus occupational therapy. Pain. 1999;83(1):77-83.
19. Rowbotham MC. Pharmacologic management of complex regional pain syndrome. Clin J Pain. 2006;22(5):425-9.
20. Kalita J, Vajpayee A, Misra UK. Comparison of prednisolone with piroxicam in complex regional pain syndrome following stroke: a randomized controlled trial. QJM. 2006;99(2):89-95.
21. Varenna M, Adami S, Rossini M, et al. Treatment of complex regional pain syndrome type I with neridronate: a randomized, double-blind, placebo-controlled study. Rheumatology (Oxford). 2013;52(3):534-42.
22. Abe Y, Iba K, Takada J, et al. Improvement of pain and regional osteoporotic changes in the foot and ankle by low-dose bisphosphonate therapy for complex regional pain syndrome type I: a case series. JM Case Rep. 2011;5:349.
23. Schwartzman RJ, Alexander GM, Grothusen JR, et al. Outpatient intravenous ketamine for the treatment of complex regional pain syndrome: a double-blind placebo controlled study. Pain. 2009;147(1-3):107-15.
24. Schwartzman RJ, Alexander GM, Grothusen JR. The use of ketamine in complex regional pain syndrome: possible mechanisms. Expert Rev Neurother. 2011;11(5):719-34.
25. Koffler SP, Hampstead BM, Irani F, et al. The neurocognitive effects of 5 day anesthetic ketamine for the treatment of refractory complex regional pain syndrome. Arch Clin Neuropsychol. 2007;22(6):719-29.
26. Goldberg ME, Torjman MC, Schwartzman RJ, et al. Pharmacodynamic profiles of ketamine (R)- and (S)- with 5-day inpatient infusion for the treatment of complex regional pain syndrome. Pain Physician. 2010;13(4):379-87.
27. van Eijs F, Geurts J, van Kleef M, et al. Predictors of pain relieving response to sympathetic blockade in complex regional pain syndrome type 1. Anesthesiology 2012;116(1):113-21.
28. Asik ZS, Orbey BC, Asik I. Sympathetic radiofrequency neurolysis for unilateral lumbar hyperhidrosis: a case report. Agri. 2008;20(3):37-9.
29. Mailis A, Furlan A. Sympathectomy for neuropathic pain. Cochrane Database Syst Rev. 2003; (2):CD002918.
30. Furlan AD, Lui PW, Mailis A. Chemical sympathectomy for neuropathic pain: does it work? Case report and systematic literature review. Clin J Pain. 2001;17(4):327-36.

13 Complex Regional Pain Syndrome—Upper Limb

Michael J Mehnert, Jeremy Simon, Matthew McAuliffe

CHIEF COMPLAINT

The patient complains of severe burning pain and swelling of the wrist and hand.

HISTORY OF PRESENT ILLNESS

A 45-year-old right-handed male presents to the outpatient clinic with complaints of severe right arm pain (Fig. 13.1). He reports that approximately 6 months ago he fell off of a ladder and went through the glass ceiling of a greenhouse 6 feet below him. The patient describes landing on an outstretched right arm. He initially was seen in the emergency room for a right forearm laceration, a scalp laceration, and wrist pain and swelling. His scalp injury was closed with staples and the right medial forearm wound was closed with sutures. Subsequently he was diagnosed with a displaced right scaphoid fracture for which he underwent surgical fixation.

On follow-up from his scaphoid fixation the patient complained of new onset epicritic, burning pain in the right forearm, wrist and hand. He reported symptoms of warmth and swelling in the right hand as well. He was prescribed pregabalin for pain control. On re-evaluation successful scaphoid fixation was appreciated on imaging; however, the patient described worsening of right arm pain with the sensation that it had "spread" to the entire forearm, wrist and hand. He described constant, severe pain in the forearm and the lateral digits of the right hand. He also stated that he had abnormal sensation in the right hand and felt as though he was "wearing a glove on just one hand". Increased erythema was reported in the right arm with swelling of the fingers and "stiffness". Pregabalin was continued at an increased dosage,

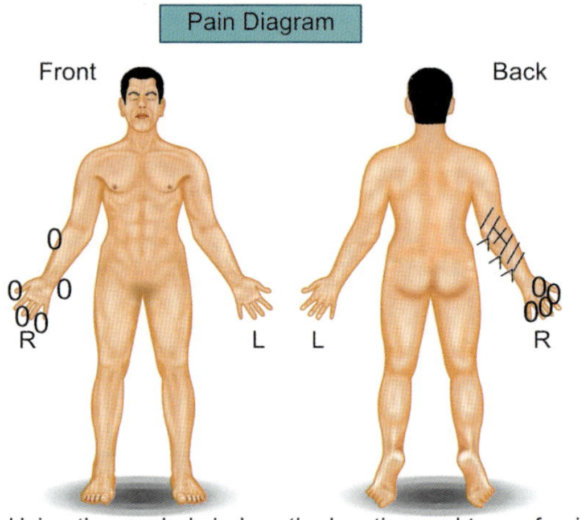

Using the symbols below, the location and type of pain sensations are marked on the diagrams. All the affected areas are included.

TYPE OF SENSATIONS	
Aching	^ ^ ^ ^ ^ ^
Sharp or stabbing	X X X X X X
Burning	//////////
Pins and needles	---------------
Numbness	0 0 0 0 0 0

Fig. 13.1: Pain diagram

and occupational therapy was prescribed for mobilization along with modalities and desensitization techniques. Electrodiagnostic testing was ordered but could not be completed due to the patients' pain and limited tolerance.

Ultimately the patient was sent for a bone scan, and findings compatible with complex regional pain syndrome (CRPS) were appreciated. No evidence of scaphoid nonunion or avascular necrosis was noted. On re-evaluation the patient continued to complain of pain and limited function of the right upper limb. He reported problems with dressing and handwriting due to pain with closing his right hand for fine motor activities. Constant, 9/10 pain was reported with hypersensitivity. No left upper limb symptoms were reported and no neck pain or shoulder/upper arm pain were described. The patient reported no prior history of similar symptoms and no fevers, chills, or other constitutional symptoms.

TREATMENTS TO DATE

Hydrocodone/APAP 5/325 mg q4 hours PRN, pregabalin 150 mg BID, occupational therapy and desensitization techniques.

PAST MEDICAL HISTORY

Gastroesophageal reflux disease, seasonal allergies.

PAST SURGICAL HISTORY

Right inguinal hernia repair.

REVIEW OF SYSTEMS

Insomnia, depressed mood, and right-hand weakness.

FAMILY HISTORY

Remarkable for type II diabetes, osteoarthritis and maternal thyroid disease.

SOCIAL HISTORY

He reports no illegal drug use and that he quit smoking 6 years ago. Rare alcohol use is described. The patient is an electrician by trade.

CURRENT MEDICATIONS

Pregabalin: 150 mg BID.

ALLERGIES

No known drug allergies.

PHYSICAL EXAMINATION

- *Height*: 5'10"
- *Weight*: 205 lbs
- Afebrile.

This is an alert, awake and cooperative male. He is in visible distress and appears anxious. Nutrition and hygiene are well-maintained. He ambulates with a normal gait and station and can do heel-and-toe walking. He cradles his right arm during most of the interview and exam.

Cervical spine exam demonstrates normal overlying skin. No tenderness is appreciated. Range of motion is full and Spurling's maneuver is negative bilaterally for any upper limb pain.

Pulses are 2+ and symmetric in the upper and lower limbs.

Reflexes are 2+ and symmetric at the biceps, triceps and brachioradialis with pain and guarding during testing on the right. Lower limb reflexes are

1+ and symmetric at the patella and Achilles. Long tract signs are absent in the lower limbs with a downgoing Babinski and in the left upper limb with a negative Hoffman's sign. This maneuver could not be tested on the right due to guarding.

Strength is 5/5 in the upper and lower limbs in all key myotomes tested on manual muscle testing, except in the right upper limb where biceps, triceps, wrist flexion and wrist extension were pain limited. He put forth minimal effort due to pain on hand intrinsic testing and active range of motion. Passive range of motion could not be performed.

A 2°C temperature difference is evident on upper limb skin temperature testing (with the right hand warmer than the left). No focal muscle atrophy is appreciated on inspection. Right scaphoid open reduction internal fixation (ORIF) scar is well-healed without erythema or drainage. Nail growth appears symmetric with no evidence of abnormal sweating or abnormal hair growth. Visible redness and swelling of all digits in the right upper limb is noted with the appearance of shiny skin over the right hand and digits.

Sensory testing to light touch and pinprick is normal in the upper and lower limbs in all key dermatomes tested, again except for the distal right upper limb where allodynia and paresthesias are appreciated with light touch in the entire hand and all digits.

IMAGING

Three-Phase Bone Scan, Right Upper Limb

Decreased uptake in the right forearm, wrist and hand with no evidence of avascular necrosis or fracture of the right scaphoid.

Right Forearm, Wrist and Hand X-rays

Pin fixation of the right scaphoid is noted without evidence of nonunion. Suspected diffuse soft-tissue swelling in the right hand is noted.

DIAGNOSIS

Complex regional pain syndrome type II involving the distal right upper limb.

DIFFERENTIAL DIAGNOSIS

Given the evaluation and testing that has already been done in this case, other diagnoses would be less likely. In fact, the criterion standard for CRPS includes ensuring that there is "no other diagnosis" that would better account for the patient's symptoms.[1] This patient seems to have recovered from an acute orthopedic injury, but has persistent and progressive symptoms. A com-petent electrodiagnostician should have been able to rule-out persistent nerve injury, however this patient could not tolerate the exam. The provided history and physical exam are not compatible with a cervical radiculopathy, though often a patient such as this would undergo a cervical spine MRI. The bone scan findings correlate with a diagnosis of CRPS and help to further rule-out nonunion, infection and other post-traumatic structural injury.

Complex Regional Pain Syndrome

Complex regional pain syndrome (previously known as reflex sympathetic dystrophy) was first described in injured soldiers under yet another name, "causalgia".[2] As discussed in the lower limb CRPS chapter, the nomenclature for sympathetic pain syndromes has evolved and is now complex regional pain syndrome, types I and II. Type II CRPS is differentiated by a documented penetrating injury or trauma, even if it is a surgical or iatrogenic event.[2] The widely accepted, recent "Budapest Criteria"[1] utilize the same model for diagnosis of CRPS I and II, and the conditions are treated as a single medical entity. The hallmark of this disease process is pain that is disproportionate to what should be expected from the injury, along with atypical symptoms that include disuse, hypersensitivity, temperature abnormalities, swelling and skin or sudomotor changes.[1] Even in cases of Type II CRPS with a documented peripheral nerve injury, the symptoms may not be isolated to that same peripheral nerve distribution, as sympathetically-mediated pain does not follow the same peripheral nerve pattern.[2,3] A triple-phase bone scan may be beneficial in diagnosing this condition, with homogenous hypoperfusion appreciated in the perfusion and blood-pool phases, along with increased periarticular uptake on the delayed images.[4,5] Changes are more prominent in early CRPS on bone scan imaging.[6] Plain films may demonstrate osteopenia as the disease persists due to disuse, with some evidence of soft tissue swelling.[6,7]

Though multiple theories as to the exact mechanism of CRPS development exist, widely accepted dogma includes a central sensitization component as well as a peripheral neural sensitization component.[3] There appears to be a role for sympathetic-mediated pain (or sympathetically maintained pain), in certain subtypes of CRPS.[8] Not all sympathetically maintained pain will meet the criteria for CRPS, and by definition response to sympathetic blocks will determine if a patient with CRPS has sympathetically-mediated pain or sympathetically-independent CRPS.[9]

TREATMENT OPTIONS

Complex regional pain syndrome treatments include palliative measures to control symptoms with modalities, medications, injection therapies and sympathectomy.[10-13] There may be a role for neuromodulation and dorsal-column stimulation for pain control as well. Many of these treatment options have been explored in the lumbar sympathetic block discussion of this book. Earlier intervention is preferred, and may result in recovery or slowed progression of symptoms.

The upper limb sympathetic innervation system includes the stellate ganglion, a structure that includes both the C7 and T1 ganglion in most patients.[14] Preganglionic fibers from the first and second thoracic spine segments travel along the ventral roots of T1 and T2 and join the sympathetic chain, synapsing at the inferior, middle or superior cervical ganglion. The inferior cervical ganglion is known as the stellate ganglion, and is generally found at the level of the first rib, spanning the C7 and T1 vertebral bodies.[15,16] All preganglionic fibers will either synapse at or pass through this ganglion.[15] Postganglionic fibers will continue on cranially to innervate neck structures. The preganglionic fibers that will innervate the upper limb originate in T2 and T8 or T9 spine segments and travel with the ventral roots of T2 to T8 to join the sympathetic chain. As they pass cephalad they also synapse at the second thoracic, first thoracic, stellate ganglion or the middle cervical ganglion. Most of these fibers travel to the anterior spinal nerves of C5-T1 and join the brachial plexus. The ganglion generally is positioned on the lateral border of the longus colli muscle.[17]

Blockade of this structure may be beneficial, particularly for newly-diagnosed CRPS in the upper limb and for certain variants or subtypes of CRPS.[18,19] The injection is now almost exclusively performed with fluoroscopic guidance and use of contrast media for safety and accuracy. Sufficient medication should be injected to bathe the C7-T1 interspace as noted above. A *successful* blockade of the ganglion (suggesting accurate delivery of anesthetic to the target stellate ganglion) will be heralded by a resulting increase in skin temperature in the upper limb on the injected side, along with increased vasodilation in the arm and temporary induction of a Horner's syndrome on the affected side. The patient should rapidly develop the classic triad of ptosis, miosis and anhidrosis with possible increased nasal congestion and skin temperature on the ipsilateral face.[20,21] The criteria for a positive diagnostic block would involve pain relief during the duration of administered anesthetic.

As with a lumbar sympathetic block, after administration of the medication immediate (occupational) therapy with range of motion, desensitization and functional retraining of the limb should be instituted.

Associated risks include bleeding, infection/abscess formation, direct neural injury, seizure, arrhythmia, syncope, death and paralysis. Potential pneumothorax and carotid or vertebral artery puncture are complications more specific to this procedure that should be discussed.[15,17] Coagulopathy is considered a contraindication if it cannot be corrected. Patients with a history of cardiac conduction block deserve careful consideration as blockade of the ganglion may affect cardiac regulation. Vital signs should be monitored prior to, during and after the procedure.

PLAN

The patient has not had relief with a therapy program and other interventions, including a trial of low-dose opiates and medications to target neuropathic pain. Given the patient's progressive pain and disability in his dominant hand, a decision was made to proceed with a right cervical stellate ganglion block with fluoroscopic guidance.

PROCEDURE NOTE

Procedure: Cervical/stellate ganglion block

INDICATIONS

Please refer to prior office notes for details. The patient is being treated for a diagnosis of complex regional pain syndrome. The patient has failed to respond to conservative measures including oral medications, modalities and physiotherapy. A decision was made to proceed with a fluoroscopically-guided cervical stellate ganglion block for diagnostic and therapeutic purposes.

The patient was informed of the risks and benefits of the procedure, as well as alternative treatments. All questions were answered prior to proceeding. The patient expressed understanding and gave informed written consent.

PREOPERATIVE DIAGNOSIS

Complex regional pain syndrome, right upper extremity.

POSTOPERATIVE DIAGNOSIS

Same

PROCEDURE PERFORMED

- Sympathetic nerve block, cervical spine (stellate ganglion block), right side
- Fluoroscopic guidance/localization.

A skin thermometer was placed on the affected limb prior to the procedure and informed consent was signed. All questions were answered, including the risks, benefits, alternative treatment options and prognosis. The risks include but are not limited to bleeding, infection, allergic reaction, nerve injury and structural damage.

The patient was taken to the fluoroscopy suite and then placed in a supine position on a fluoroscopy table with a shoulder roll in place with the cervical spine in a slightly extended position, as much as tolerated. The affected side was prepped with antiseptic solution and draped in the usual sterile fashion. Vital signs and oxygen saturation were monitored pre- and periprocedurally. Cardiac monitoring revealed normal sinus rhythm.

The cricoid cartilage was palpated and the figertips were moved laterally, displacing the sterno-cleidomastoid and the carotid sheath laterally. Chassaignac's tubercle, the transverse process of the sixth cervical vertebra, was identified under fluoroscopic guidance, palpated, and then isolated between two palpating fingertips. Once the carotid sheath was out of the way, a 22-gauge needle was inserted perpendicularly to all planes and placed on the anterior lateral border of the C-6 vertebral body. Aspiration was then attempted. After aspiration was negative for return of blood or other fluid, 3–5 mL of nonionic radio-opaque contrast media were injected (Figs 13.2 and 13.3) and noted to flow over the lateral borders of the ipsilateral cervical vertebral bodies, thus covering the stellate ganglion. Live fluoroscopy was utilized to ensure the absence of vascular flow of contrast. A test dose of 0.5 mL of 1% lidocaine was then injected, and the patient was monitored for 60–90 seconds to ensure no adverse effects to suggest intravascular injection. Next, a solution of 10 mL of marcaine 0.25% in aliquots of 2 mL with negative aspirations between injections was administered, with intermittent fluoroscopy utilized to ensure further washout of the contrast. The patient tolerated the procedure well without any evidence of complications or problems. Post-procedure they experienced the following:

Evidence of a Horner's sign after the block was established: YES

Pain relief: 80%

Skin temperature change was greater than 10 degrees.

The patient tolerated the procedure well and was discharged after an appropriate period of observation. If there are any complications, the patient was instructed to call us. The patient is to follow-up with the physician as noted above within 2–3 weeks.

The patient was instructed to apply ice over the injection site for 10–15 minutes for the next 24–48 hours. A postprocedure instruction sheet was given.

STELLATE GANGLION BLOCK (FIGS 13.2 AND 13.3)

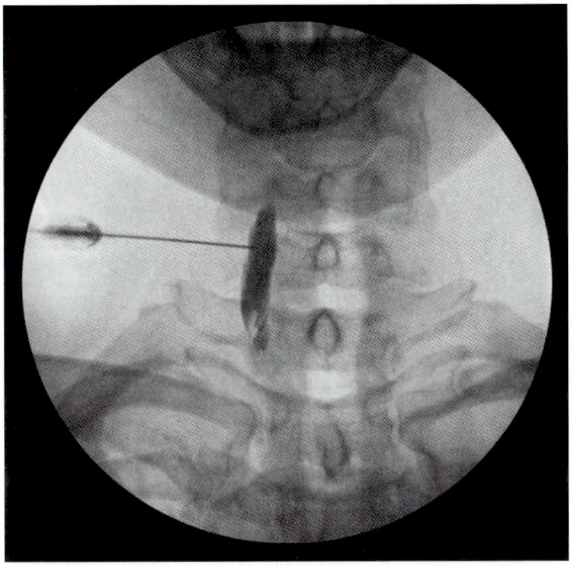

Fig. 13.2

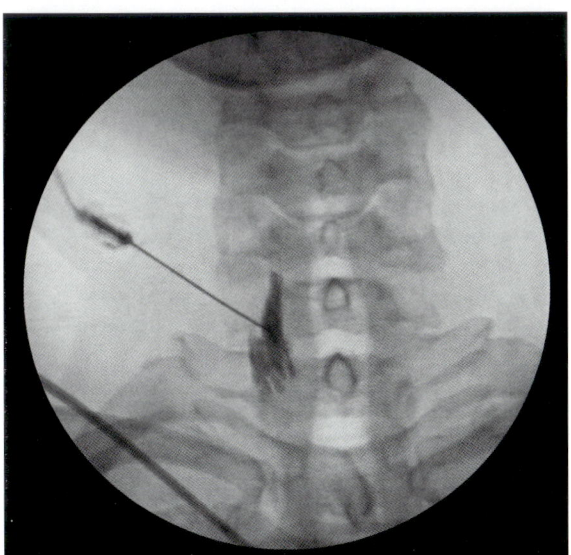

Fig. 13.3

Figs 13.2 and 13.3: Anterior posterior views of a right stellate ganglion block after contrast administration

REFERENCES

1. Harden RN, Bruehl S, Stanton-Hicks M, et al. Proposed new diagnostic criteria for complex regional pain syndrome. Pain Med. 2007;8(4):326-31.
2. Harden RN, Oaklander AL, Burton AW, et al. Complex regional pain syndrome: practical diagnostic and treatment guidelines, 4th edition. Pain Med. 2013;14:180-229.
3. Marinus J, Moseley GL, Birklein F, et al. Clinical features and pathophysiology of complex regional pain syndrome. Lancet Neurol. 2011;10(7):637-48.
4. Mailis A. How are bone scans used in the diagnosis and treatment of CRPS? RSDSA Review. 2005;18:11.
5. Intenzo CM, Kim SM, Capuzzi DM. The role of nuclear medicine in the evaluation of complex regional pain syndrome type I. Clin Nucl Med. 2005;30(6):400-7.
6. Schurmann M, Zaspel J, Lohr P, et al. Imaging in early posttraumatic complex regional pain syndrome: a comparison of diagnostic methods. Clin J Pain. 2007; 23(5):449-57.
7. Cappello ZJ, Kasdan ML, Louis DS. Meta-analysis of imaging techniques for the diagnosis of complex regional pain syndrome type I. J Hand Surg. 2012;37(2):288-96.
8. Stanton-Hicks M, Janig W, Hassenbusch S, et al. Reflex sympathetic dystrophy: changing concepts and taxonomy. Pain 1995;63(1):127-33.
9. Raja SN, Treede RD, Davis KD, et al. Systemic alpha-adrenergic blockade with phentolamine: a diagnostic test for sympathetically maintained pain. Anesthesiology. 1991;74(4):691-8.
10. Rowbotham MC. Pharmacologic management of complex regional pain syndrome. Clin J Pain. 2006;22(5):425-9.
11. Mailis A, Furlan A. Sympathectomy for neuropathic pain. Cochrane database Syst Rev. 2003; (7):CD002918.
12. Braus DF, Krauss JK, Strobel J. The shoulder-hand syndrome after stroke: a prospective clinical trial. Ann Neurol. 1994;36(5):728-33.
13. Oerlemans HM, Goris JA, de Boo T, et al. Do physical therapy and occupational therapy reduce the impairment percentage in reflex sympathetic dystrophy? Am J Phys Med Rehabil/Assoc Acad Physiatr. 1999;78:533-9.
14. Benzon HT Raja SN, Molloy RE, et al. Essentials of Pain Medicine and Regional Anesthesia, 2nd edition. Philadelphia, PA: Elsevier; 2005.
15. Haspeslagh S VKM. Sympathetic System. Philadelphia, PA: Saunders Elsevier; 2008.
16. Fox M. Stellate ganglion block. Philadelphia, PA: Elsevier-Saunders; 2013.
17. Hogan QH, Erickson SJ. MR imaging of the stellate ganglion: normal appearance. AJR Am J Roentgenol. 1992;158(3):655-9.
18. Blain A 3rd. Cervical sympathetic and stellate ganglion block in apoplexy; preliminary note on indications and technique. Alexander Blain Hosp Bull. 1949;8(1):42-6.
19. van Eijs F, Stanton-Hicks M, Van Zundert J, et al. Evidence-based interventional pain medicine according to clinical diagnoses. 16. Complex regional pain syndrome. Pain Pract. 2011;11(1):70-87.
20. Abdi S, Zhou Y, Patel N, et al. A new and easy technique to block the stellate ganglion. Pain Physician. 2004;7(3):327-31.
21. van Eijs F, Geurts J, van Kleef M, et al. Predictors of pain relieving response to sympathetic blockade in complex regional pain syndrome type 1. Anesthesiology. 2012;116(1):113-21.

14 Dural Puncture Headache

Jeremy Simon

CHIEF COMPLAINT

The patient complains of severe headache.

HISTORY OF PRESENT ILLNESS

This patient is a 52-year-old female with a past medical history significant for 10 years of gradually increasing lower back and bilateral buttock pain. She underwent 2 nonfluoroscopically-guided L5-S1 interlaminar epidural steroid injections approximately 2 weeks apart as part of a "series of three". The first of these injections was performed 3 weeks ago, the second less than 1 week ago. She is unsure if the first injection helped and had no significant side effects or complaints. Upon awakening the following day after the second injection, she experienced a severe headache. It has persisted and not improved over the last 2 days. She rates the pain a 10/10 with standing or sitting and a 4/10 with lying flat. It is located in the temples, associated with nausea and dizziness. She has never had a headache like this before. It is significantly worse with sitting upright, standing, and relieved somewhat with lying flat. There are no fevers, chills or night sweats. She has not started any new medications and the headache is not responsive to ibuprofen 800 mg PO TID. There are no new sensory or motor symptoms.

PAST MEDICAL HISTORY

None

PAST SURGICAL HISTORY

None

REVIEW OF SYSTEMS

Positive for headache, photophobia, nausea, lower back and buttock pain

FAMILY HISTORY

Hypertension

SOCIAL HISTORY

Denies tobacco, alcohol or illegal drugs. Manager of a retail store. Has not worked since onset of symptoms. No worker's compensation claims.

CURRENT MEDICATIONS

Ibuprofen: 800 mg TID, multivitamin

ALLERGIES

None

PHYSICAL EXAMINATION

- *BP*: 140/90 mm Hg
- *Pulse*: 90/minute
- *Respirations*: 14/minute
- *Height*: 5'4"
- *Weight*: 100 lbs

General Appearance

Pleasant, cooperative, looks stated age*, in obvious distress, lying on exam table flat on her back with knees bent.*

Gait and tandem gait stable, with *slight forward flexion*. Romberg sign is negative. Able to heel walk and toe walk without difficulty. Pulses are 2+ in the radial and dorsalis pedis arteries. Babinski testing reveals downgoing toes bilaterally. Slump test and supine straight leg raised to 90° are negative bilaterally. Negative femoral nerve stretch test bilaterally. No palpable step-off in the lumbar spine. No tenderness over the lumbar spinous processes. No palpable scoliotic curve. *There is palpable muscle spasm in the lumbar paraspinals and tenderness*. Patrick's test is negative bilaterally. Internal rotation of the hips does not cause pain. No tenderness to palpation over the bilateral trochanteric bursae. Negative Gaenslen's sign, negative Thomas test, negative Ober's test bilaterally. No tenderness over the sacroiliac joints. Manual muscle testing in the lower limbs reveals 5/5 bilateral hip flexors, quadriceps, tibialis anterior, extensor hallucis longus and gastrocsoleus. Sensory examination to light touch and pinprick is normal in the lower extremity dermatomes. Proprioception is intact at the great toes bilaterally. Normal muscle tone. Reflexes are 2+ in patellae, medial hamstrings and Achilles tendons. No ankle clonus bilaterally. *Lumbar range of motion is reduced in extension and the end limits of flexion. There is reproduction of typical pain with extension and extension/rotation to the right.* Posterior-anterior pressure over the L4-5 and L5-S1 segments on the right cause reproduction of pain.

Cranial nerves II-XII were intact. *Upright posture causes severe headache and nausea.*

IMAGING

Magnetic resonance imaging lumbar spine from 2 months ago demonstrates moderately severe spinal stenosis at L4-5, facet arthropathy at L4-5 and L5-S1.

DIAGNOSIS

Post-dural puncture headache (PDPH) (spinal headache).

DISCUSSION

Post-dural puncture headache most likely occurs as result of a needle piercing the dura mater covering the thecal sac and a resultant leakage of spinal fluid.[1] This results in reduced intracranial pressure and a postural headache.[1,2] Why the headache occurs is postulated to be a result of the loss of cushion of the meninges through loss of cerebrospinal fluid (CSF) through the hole created by the needle.[3,4]

The characteristics of PDPH are typically bilateral and temporal and may occur anywhere from immediately following or up to 12 days after a lumbar puncture.[3] It is classically worse with upright posture. They are often self-limited, but may result in significant morbidity including nausea, vomiting and neck pain.[3] Patients experiencing these symptoms may visit the emergency room, undergo diagnostic testing and take analgesic medications and miss work, resulting in significant direct and indirect medical costs.

Risk factors reported for the development of PDPH include female gender, younger age and low body mass index.[5,6] A smaller-size needle has also shown to play a role in reduction of the development of PDPH.[7] The use of fluoroscopy in epidural steroid injections should also play a role reducing risk of PDPH, as well as other potential serious complications.[8,9] One study recently showed a lower incidence of PDPH in cigarette smokers.[10] Certainly, this is not meant to encourage smoking, but in the diagnosis of PDPH in our patient, the low BMI, female gender, blind-epidurals performed, characteristics of the headache (positional, frontal/temporal) and the non-smoking status paint an obvious clinical picture.

Fluoroscopy for placement of epidural steroid injections is not universally utilized. Studies have shown inaccurate injection in 8–30% of nonfluoroscopically-guided lumbar epidural steroid injections[11] and up to 53% in blind cervical epidural steroid injections.[12] Many practitioners also perform epidurals in a "series" despite the lack of evidence in a clear benefit of repetition.

TREATMENT

Most PDPHs will resolve on their own.[13] Conservative treatment consists of increasing oral fluid intake, caffeine and nonsteroidal anti-inflammatory medications. Caffeine has shown efficacy for treating this condition over placebo.[14] Bed rest is often recommended and shown to have mixed results.[15,16]

An epidural blood patch can be considered for recalcitrant headache resulting from dural puncture. This procedure involves injecting the patient's blood into the epidural space, with or without fluoroscopic guidance (Figs 14.1 and 14.2). The use of fluoroscopy in this procedure improves the accuracy and are likely safer than using a blind approach.[17]

The success rate is reported to be between 70% and 100%.[13,18] The proposed mechanism of action is to form a clot over the hole in the dura and thus stop the CSF from leaking.[3] The volume of blood injected may range from 7 mL to 30 mL.[13] Risks of the procedure include compressive epidural hematoma, meningitis, dural puncture, death, subdural hematoma,[19,20] stroke,[21] blindness, arachnoiditis,[22] fever,[23] and scar formation.

This patient underwent an epidural blood patch and her symptoms completely resolved in 2 days.

Sample Dictation

Informed consent was signed prior to the procedure. The risks, benefits, alternative treatment options, prognosis and questions were discussed. The risks include, but not limited to, epidural hematoma, meningitis, dural puncture, new or worsening pain, subdural hematoma, arachnoiditis, fever, scar formation and nerve damage.

The patient was then prepped and draped in a sterile fashion in the prone position. Vital signs and oxygen saturation were monitored throughout the procedure.

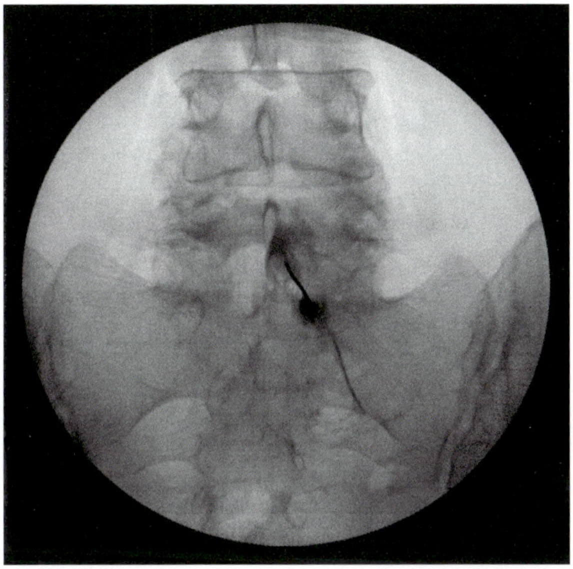

Fig 14.1: Anterior and posterior view of contrast extending into the epidural space

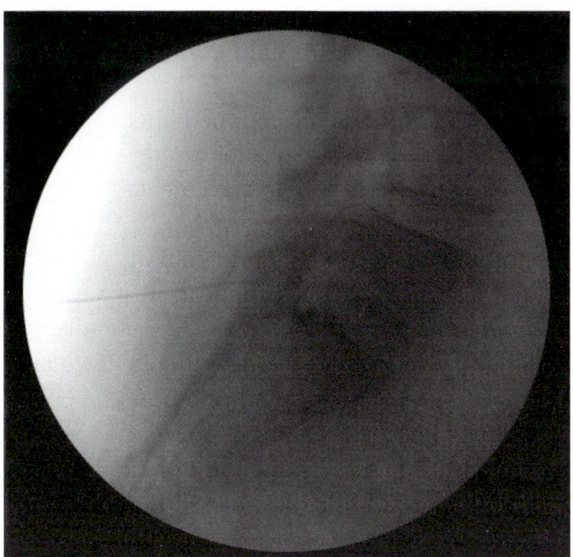

Fig 14.2: Lateral view with contrast extending into the epidural space

Around 10–20 cc of the patient's blood was withdrawn in a sterile fashion via an intravenous needle placed at the start of the procedure.

The C-arm was positioned so that an AP view of the L5-S1 interlaminar space was visualized. The soft tissues overlying the area were infiltrated with 3 cc of 1% lidocaine without epinephrine. An 18-gauge Tuohy needle was inserted under intermittent fluoroscopy to just superior to the inferior lamina via a paramedian approach. A lateral image was then obtained and the needle advanced to just superficial to the spinolaminar line. The epidural space was localized with a loss of resistance technique. After negative aspiration for blood or CSF, a 1 cc volume of nonionic iodinated contrast was injected and flow of contrast was noted. Radiographs were obtained for documentation purposes. Initially, 2 cc of 1% lidocaine was injected as a "test dose". No adverse reaction was noted. The patient's autologous blood was then administered slowly through the needle. After the blood was injected, the needle was flushed with 1% lidocaine and removed. A bandage was placed over the injection site. The patient laid prone for an additional minute and then was taken to the recovery area.

REFERENCES

1. Serpell MG, Rawal N. Headaches after diagnostic dural punctures. BMJ. 2000;321(7267):973-4.
2. Grant R, Condon B, Hart I, et al. Changes in intracranial CSF volume after lumbar puncture and their relationship to post-LP headache. J Neurol Neurosurg Psychiatry. 1991;54(5):440-2.
3. Ahmed SV, Jayawarna C, Jude E. Post lumbar puncture headache: diagnosis and management. Postgrad Med J. 2006;82(973):713-6.
4. Hatfalvi BI. Postulated mechanisms for postdural puncture headache and review of laboratory models. Clinical experience. Reg Anesth. 1995;20(4): 329-36.
5. Kuntz KM, Kokmen E, Stevens JC, et al. Post-lumbar puncture headaches: experience in 501 consecutive procedures. Neurology. 1992;42(10):1884-7.
6. Leibold RA, Yealy DM, Coppola M, et al. Post-dural-puncture headache: characteristics, management, and prevention. Ann Emerg Med. 1993; 22(12): 1863-70.
7. Stendell L, Fomsgaard JS, Olsen KS. There is room for improvement in the prevention and treatment of headache after lumbar puncture. Dan Med J. 2012;59(7):A4483.
8. Johnson BA. Image-guided epidural injections. Neuroimaging Clin N Am. 2000;10(3):479-91.
9. Furman MB, O'Brien EM, Zgleszewski TM. Incidence of intravascular penetration in transforaminal lumbosacral epidural steroid injections. Spine. 2000;25(20):2628-32.
10. Dodge HS, Ekhator NN, Jefferson-Wilson L, et al. Cigarette smokers have reduced risk for post-dural puncture headache. Pain Physician. 2013;16(1): E25-30.
11. Bartynski WS, Grahovac SZ, Rothfus WE. Incorrect needle position during lumbar epidural steroid administration: inaccuracy of loss of air pressure resistance and requirement of fluoroscopy and epidurography during needle insertion. AJNR Am J Neuroradiol. 2005;26:502-5.
12. Stojanovic MP, Vu TN, Caneris O, et al. The role of fluoroscopy in cervical epidural steroid injections: an analysis of contrast dispersal patterns. Spine. 2002;27(5):509-14.

13. Turnbull DK, Shepherd DB. Post-dural puncture headache: pathogenesis, prevention and treatment. Br J Anaesth. 2003;91(5):718-29.
14. Basurto Ona X, Martinez Garcia L, Sola I, et al. Drug therapy for treating post-dural puncture headache. Cochrane Database Syst Rev. 2011;(8):CD007887.
15. Allen C, Glasziou P, Del Mar C. Bed rest: a potentially harmful treatment needing more careful evaluation. Lancet. 1999;354(9186):1229-33.
16. Teece S, Crawford I. Towards evidence based emergency medicine: best BETs from the Manchester Royal Infirmary. Bed rest after lumbar puncture. Emerg Med J. Emerg Med J. 2002;19(5):432-3.
17. Cho KI, Moon HS, Jeon HJ, et al. Spontaneous intracranial hypotension: efficacy of radiologic targeting vs blind blood patch. Neurology. 2011;76(13):1139-44.
18. Kawaguchi M, Hashizume K, Watanabe K, et al. Fluoroscopically guided epidural blood patch in patients with postdural puncture headache after spinal and epidural anesthesia. J Anesth. 2011;25(3):450-3.
19. Schott M, Gehrke A, Gaab M, et al. [Subdural hematoma after dural puncture: fateful complication of epidural anesthesia]. Anaesthesist. 2013;62(5):392-5.
20. Verduzco LA, Atlas SW, Riley ET. Subdural hematoma after an epidural blood patch. Int J Obstet Anesth. 2012;21(2):189-92.
21. Ng MD, Manikappa S. Postpartum seizure and ischaemic stroke following dural puncture and epidural blood patch. Anaesth Intensive Care. 2012;40(2):347-51.
22. Al Maach N, Vogels OJ, Bollen TL, et al. Arachnoiditis and communicating hydrocephalus as a complication of epidural blood patch. J Neurol. 2010; 257(4):672-3.
23. Hunyady AI, Anderson CT, Kuratani JD, et al. Fever following an Epidural Blood Patch in a Child. Case Rep Anesthesiol. 2012;2012:753875.

15 Adverse Reactions to Medications

Jeremy Simon

CHIEF COMPLAINT

Low back and left lower extremity pain.

HISTORY OF PRESENT ILLNESS

A 26-year-old male with no significant medical history was moving out of his medical school apartment and lifted a couch 10 weeks ago. He was taking it down the steps with his fiancé and maneuvering in the hallway. He almost dropped it, twisted and felt a "pop" in the left side of his low back. He felt immediate pain, 10/10, followed by pain radiating to the left lower limb. Now the leg pain is 9/10 and the back pain 6/10, worse with sitting and bending, better with standing with his left leg extended. It is dull and aching in the left low back, sharp in the left buttock and electric-like and sharp in the posterior left thigh, calf and lateral left foot. There are associated paresthesias in the left outer foot and fifth toe. He notices slight weakness. The pain is constant. He has tried ibuprofen 800 mg PO TID, cyclobenzaprine 10 mg PO TID, heat/ice, and five sessions of physical therapy with very little benefit. He started internship in 4 weeks.

PAST MEDICAL HISTORY

None

PAST SURGICAL HISTORY

None

REVIEW OF SYSTEMS

Positive for above otherwise negative.

FAMILY HISTORY

Diabetes type II

SOCIAL HISTORY

Denies tobacco or illegal drugs, drinks occasional alcohol. Finished medical school and is starting internship in general surgery.

CURRENT MEDICATIONS

None (discontinued 2 weeks ago due to lack of benefit).

ALLERGIES

No known drug allergies

PHYSICAL EXAMINATION

- *Height*: 6'0"
- *Weight*: 180 lbs
- *BP*: 110/70 mm Hg
- *Pulse*: 70/minute

General Appearance

Pleasant, cooperative, alert and oriented, no acute distress.
Inspection: No asymmetry, no evidence of scoliosis.
Gait: nonantalgic, able to ambulate on heels, and tandem without difficulty, *difficulty with toe walking.*
Range of motion: Limitations in flexion with more pain reproduction in flexion than extension.

Neurological

Strength: Manual muscle testing 5/5 with exception of *left plantar flexion and flexor hallucis longus 4+/5.*
Sensation: *Decreased light touch and pinprick over lateral aspect of foot on the left.*

Reflexes: Symmetrical bilateral patellae and Achilles reflex.
Provocative: *Straight leg raise and sitting dural tension signs positive on the left.*
Musculoskeletal: Hip internal and external with pain-free normal range of motion, FABER negative bilaterally.

IMAGING

X-rays: Patient brings lumbar X-rays from his family physician AP/lateral/oblique/flexion and extension showing normal segmentation, no spondylolisthesis, spondylolysis and normal disc height.

Magnetic resonance imaging lumbar spine demonstrates a moderate size left paracentral disc extrusion at L5-S1 in contact with the left S1 nerve root.

DIAGNOSIS

Acute left S1 radiculopathy secondary to L5-S1 disc herniation.

Plan

It was recommended for this patient to undergo a left S1 transforaminal epidural steroid injection under fluoroscopy due to the severe limb greater than back pain and his failure of conservative treatment at 10 weeks. He is also to start internship and wants the opportunity to reduce his pain quickly. Surgical options of microdiscectomy were also discussed and a referral was given for an orthopedic spine surgeon if the conservative treatments were to fail.

Method of Procedure

Left S1 transforaminal epidural steroid injection under fluoroscopy.

Informed consent was signed and all questions were answered prior to procedure. The risks, benefits and alternative treatment options were explained. The risks include, but are not limited to, infections, epidural hematoma, nerve damage, spinal cord infarction, paralysis, spinal headache, new or worsening pain, and scar formation. The patient's vital signs and oxygen saturation were monitored prior, during and after the procedure.

The C-arm was positioned so that an AP view of the S1 foramen was visualized. The soft tissues and skin were anesthetized with 3 cc of 1% lidocaine without epinephrine. A 22-gauge spinal needle was inserted toward the posterior aspect of the sacrum just lateral and inferior to the S1 pedicle. The needle was advanced under a lateral projection into the sacral canal at the S1-2 level.

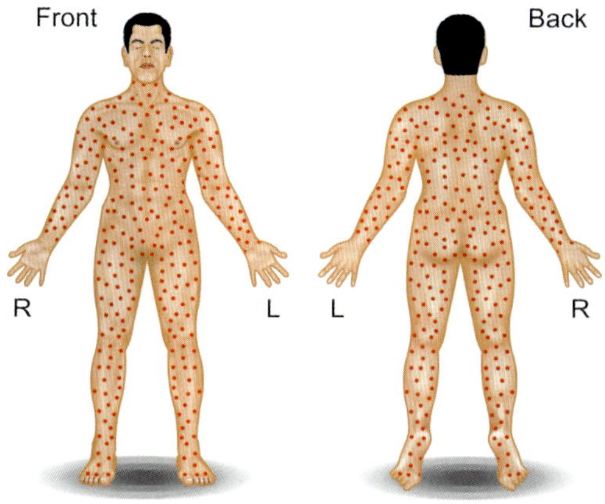

Fig. 15.1: Patient symptom diagram. Patient describes a whole body rash with itching

After negative aspirate for blood or CSF, approximately a total volume of 1 cc of nonionic contrast was injected and flow of contrast was noted. Radiographs were obtained for documentation purposes. An injectate of 4 cc consisting of 2 cc of 6 mg/cc betamethasone, 1 cc of 1% lidocaine without epinephrine and the remainder of normal saline was then injected.

Following the procedure, the patient was taken to the recovery area and vital signs were repeated.

Postprocedure: As the discharge instructions were discussed approximately 10 minutes after the procedure, the patient felt itching in the throat and a raised rash on the trunk began to develop. There was also a "full feeling" in the tongue and mouth (Fig. 15.1).

ADDITIONAL DIAGNOSIS

Anaphylactic reaction, likely secondary to medication administered during epidural steroid injection.

Plan

The patient was placed on the cardiac monitor and given a bolus of 50 mg of IV diphenhydramine and 0.5 mg IM epinephrine. Emergency medical services (EMS) were called, as well. Oxygen via mask was placed at 10 L/minute and vital signs were repeated. The patient's heart rate and blood pressure were 100 bpm and 140/90 mm Hg. The patient's oxygen saturation remained at 98% on masked oxygen. His rash began to fade in 5 minutes and he was breathing better and less labored when EMS arrived.

DISCUSSION

Anaphylactic and pseudo-anaphylactic reactions appear as clinically identical entities.[1] The two are distinguished only by whether or not antibodies are involved in the mediation of histamine release.[1] Prior exposure to an antigen is necessary for a true anaphylactic reaction. When the antigen is reintroduced, the antigen binds to IgE or IgG, which then binds to a mast cell and basophils and releases histamine, leukotrienes, prostaglandins, and other chemicals causing a systemic-anaphylactic reaction.[1]

The possibility of severe anaphylactic reaction is one that the interventionist need be prepared for in the injection suite. This patient developed the rapid onset of shortness of breath, angioedema and urticaria while in the recovery room. All patients should be consented for the possibility of an anaphylactic reaction for an interventional spine procedure and equipment should be readily available was the need to arise.

While the medications utilized during an epidural steroid injection are minimal, recognition of the potential for any of them to cause an allergic reaction should be noted. Allergies to local anesthetics have been documented.[2,3] Side effects should be differentiated from true allergies as many patients will report increased heart rate with epinephrine containing anesthetics used in dental and other procedures.

Reports of allergy to steroid compounds are also documented.[4] The symptoms should also be clarified as common side effects from steroids may be misinterpreted as allergy. The common side effects include a facial or truncal flushing reaction, dizziness, headache, pruritus, increased blood sugar in diabetics, menstrual cycle changes, "jitteriness" and insomnia.[3] Mood changes and rarely psychosis may also occur.[5,6]

The use of contrast agents is also a significant potential source of allergy. Most of the contrast agents utilized in epidural steroid injections are iodine-containing. While the newer agents are nonionic, closer to physiologic osmolality and contain a smaller amount of free-iodine, patients with a known iodine allergy should be premedicated with anti-histamines, both H1 and H2 blockers, and steroid.[7] Some practitioners advocate utilizing gadolinium in cases of severe allergy,[8] although this material is not as radiodense and subtle vascular flow may be missed. Cases of allergy to gadodiamide have also been reported.[9] While not as common, allergies to topical iodine-povidine and chlorhexidine have been reported, as well.[10-14]

Treatment of the anaphylactic reaction should begin immediately. Autoinjectors of epinephrine should be readily available.[15] Epinephrine has been shown to be the most effective treatment in the treatment of anaphylaxis.[15,16] Supportive treatment with supplemental oxygen should also be provided. Emergent care also includes administration of antihistamine, typically diphenhydramine, an H2 blocker such as ranitidine and steroids. Resuscitation equipment should be available in the procedure suite as severe anaphylactic reactions may result in cardiac and pulmonary arrest. EMS should be called immediately if the reaction is occurring as a precaution.

After the patient is stabilized and the reaction is abated, a consultation with an allergy specialist is recommended. Skin prick or patch testing may provide the answer as to which agent or agents caused the anaphylactic reaction.[17]

REFERENCES

1. Ring J, Behrendt H, de Weck A. History and classification of anaphylax's. Chen Immunol Allergy. 2010;95:1-11.
2. Caron AB. Allergy to multiple local anesthetics. Allergy and asthma proceedings: the official journal of regional and state allergy societies. 2007;28:600-1.
3. Goodman BS, Posecion LW, Mallempati S, et al. Complications and pitfalls of lumbar interlaminar and transforaminal epidural injections. Curr Rev Musculoskelet Med. 2008;1(3-4):212-22.
4. Kamm GL, Hagmeyer KO. Allergic-type reactions to corticosteroids. Ann Pharmacother. 1999;33(4):451-60.
5. Milgrom H, Bender BG. Psychologic side effects of therapy with corticosteroids. Am Rev Respir Dis. 1993;147(2):471-3.
6. Brown ES, Khan DA, Nejtek VA. The psychiatric side effects of corticosteroids. Ann Allergy Asthma Immunol. 1999;83(6 Pt 1):495-503.
7. Meth MJ, Maibach HI. Current understanding of contrast media reactions and implications for clinical management. Drug Saf. 2006;29(2):133-41.
8. Safriel Y, Ali M, Hayt M, et al. Gadolinium use in spine procedures for patients with allergy to iodinated contrast-experience of 127 procedures. AJNR Am J Neuroradiol. 2006;27(6):1194-7.
9. O'Donnell CJ, Cano WG. Allergic reactions to gadodiamide following interventional spinal procedures: a report of 4 cases. Arch Phys Med Rehabil. 2007;88(11):1465-7.
10. Aliagaoglu C, Turan H, Uslu E, et al. Iododerma following topical povidone-iodine application. Cutan Ocul Toxicol. 2013.
11. Cheng CE, Kroshinsky D. Iatrogenic skin injury in hospitalized patients. Clin Dermatol. 2011;29(6):622-32.
12. Masse M, Falanga V, Zhou LH. Use of topical povidone-iodine resulting in an iododerma-like eruption. J Dermatol.2008;35(11):744-7.
13. Keni NN, Aras MA, Chitre V. Chlorhexidine allergy due to topical application. Indian J Dent Res. 2012;23(5):674-6.
14. Liippo J, Kousa P, Lammintausta K. The relevance of chlorhexidine contact allergy. Contact Dermatitis. 2011;64(4):229-34.

15. Simons FE. Anaphylaxis. J Allergy Clin Immunol. 2010;125(2 Suppl):S161-181.
16. Simons FE, Ardusso LR, Bilo MB, et al. 2012 Update: World Allergy Organization Guidelines for the assessment and management of anaphylaxis. Curr Opin Allergy Clin Immunol. 2012;12(4):389-99.
17. Rive CM, Bourke J, Phillips EJ. Testing for drug hypersensitivity syndromes. Clin Biochem Rev. 2013;34(1):15-38.

Discogenic Low Back Pain/ Lumbar Disc Herniation without Radiculopathy

16

Jeremy Simon, Zachary Broyer, Theodore Conliffe

CHIEF COMPLAINT

The patient complains of constant lower back and buttock pain (Fig. 16.1).

HISTORY OF PRESENT ILLNESS

This patient is a 45-year-old construction worker with a past medical history significant for two previous lumbar sprain/strain injuries at work over the last 6 years. These episodes resolved after approximately 3–4 weeks with the help of nonsteroidal anti-inflammatory medications and relative rest. Three months ago, he was lifting several bags of concrete at work and felt a "pop" in his lower back. He had immediate lower back pain, sharp in nature. The pain has become constant with intermittent radiation to the bilateral buttocks, but not all the way down the legs. There is a constant ache and he rates the pain an average of 6/10, worse with sitting, bending, twisting and standing for extended periods of time. There is pain with bowel movements, coughing and sneezing. Lying flat and arching his back helps slightly. Nonsteroidal anti-inflammatory medications and cyclobenzaprine have not helped substantially. The patient tells you he wants to go back to work, but the pain is preventing him from going back and enjoying life. He denies associated numbness, tingling, or weakness in the lower extremities and there is no saddle anesthesia. He denies fevers, chills or night sweats, unintentional weight loss or weight gain, or hip pain. This is a worker's compensation claim.

Treatments to date include anti-inflammatory medications, muscle relaxers, eight sessions of physical therapy, one L5-S1 interlaminar epidural steroid injection and one bilateral S1 transforaminal epidural steroid injection without significant relief.

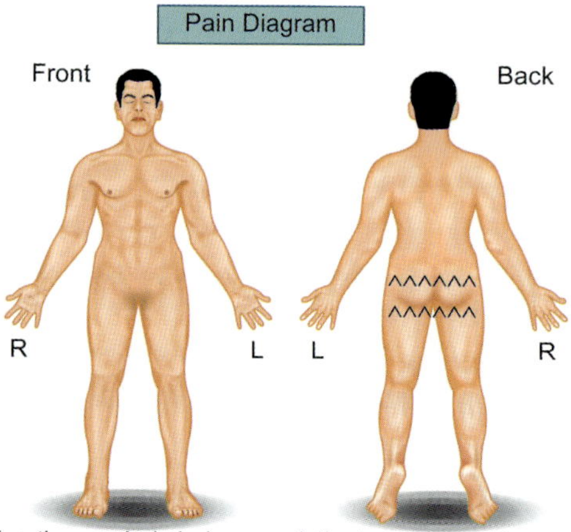

Using the symbols below, mark the location and type of pain on the diagram on the left. Include all affected areas.

TYPE OF SENSATIONS

Aching	^ ^ ^ ^ ^ ^
Sharp or stabbing	X X X X X X
Burning	//////////
Pins and needles	--------------
Numbness	0 0 0 0 0 0

Fig. 16.1: Pain diagram

PAST MEDICAL HISTORY

As above

PAST SURGICAL HISTORY

Wisdom teeth removed

REVIEW OF SYSTEMS

As above otherwise negative

FAMILY HISTORY

Parents alive with hypertension

SOCIAL HISTORY

Smokes half pack of cigarettes a day for 20 years, occasional alcohol, no illicit drugs. He works as a construction laborer, but is currently out of work due to pain since this injury. There is no light duty.

CURRENT MEDICATIONS

Cyclobenzaprine 10 mg PO BID PRN, naprosyn 500 mg PO BID

ALLERGIES

None

PHYSICAL EXAMINATION

- *Height*: 6'0"
- *Weight*: 190 lbs
- *Blood pressure*: 120/70 mm Hg
- *Pulse*: 62/minute

General Appearance

Pleasant, cooperative, alert and oriented, in obvious discomfort

Inspection

No asymmetry, no evidence of scoliosis

Gait

Nonantalgic, able to ambulate on heels, toes and tandem without difficulty

Range of Motion

Pain reproduction in flexion and less pain with extension

Neurological

Strength: Manual muscle testing 5/5 in the bilateral lower limbs
Sensation: Intact to light touch and pin prick in the bilateral lower limbs
Reflexes: Symmetrical bilateral patellae and Achilles reflex
Provocative: Straight leg raise and sitting dural tension signs negative; *however, there is reproduction of pain in the buttocks and back bilaterally*
Musculoskeletal: Hip internal and external with pain-free normal range of motion, FABER negative bilaterally

Waddell's signs are negative.

IMAGING

Lumbar Spine X-Rays

Normal segmentation. No scoliosis. No evidence for fractures or spondylolithesis. Reduced disc-space height is noted at L5-S1.

Lumbar Spine Magnetic Resonance Imaging without Gadolinium

Mild disc space narrowing at L4-5 and moderate disc narrowing at L5-S1. There is an area of increased signal intensity on T2-weighted images in the posterior aspect of the L5-S1 disc and a central protrusion.

DIAGNOSIS

Likely discogenic low back pain secondary to annular tear at L5-S1.

Plan

The patient was counseled on discogenic lower back pain. It was explained that the treatments for this entity are not as predictably successful as with disc herniations associated with mostly limb pain. Options for treatment were discussed as well as the benign nature of his pain (i.e. that it is not life-threatening). Recommendations were made for continued physical therapy, avoidance of aggravating factors, and pain-coping strategies. The patient was also counseled to stop smoking as there is a negative association with smoking and pain, as well as disc healing.[1] Surgical options were discussed as well as the possibility of discography should he wish to pursue this option. The patient was placed on light duty work and a functional capacity evaluation was considered. The patient wished to discuss the options with his wife and to return for assessment in 4 weeks.

The patient returned for follow-up 4 weeks later with his wife. They both expressed that the pain had become unbearable and was affecting almost every aspect of their lives. They could not have sexual intercourse due to the severity of the pain. They requested a surgical consultation (Fig. 16.2). It was explained to the patient that prior to the surgical consultation, confirmation of the diagnosis need be made by a provocative lumbar discogram. The risks, benefits, and alternative treatment options were discussed with them and they expressed understanding.

Lumbar Provocative Discography Method of Procedure

Informed consent for the procedure was obtained. The risks, benefits and alternative options were discussed. The risks include, but are not limited to, death, paralysis, allergic reaction, syncope, arrhythmia, cardiac or respiratory arrest, spinal cord injury, worse pain, scar formation, bleeding, epidural hematoma and infection. The patient was prepped and draped in a sterile fashion while in the prone position. All vital signs and oxygen saturation were monitored prior to, during, and after the procedure. All personnel in the operating room were wearing masks, head and foot protection to reduce the

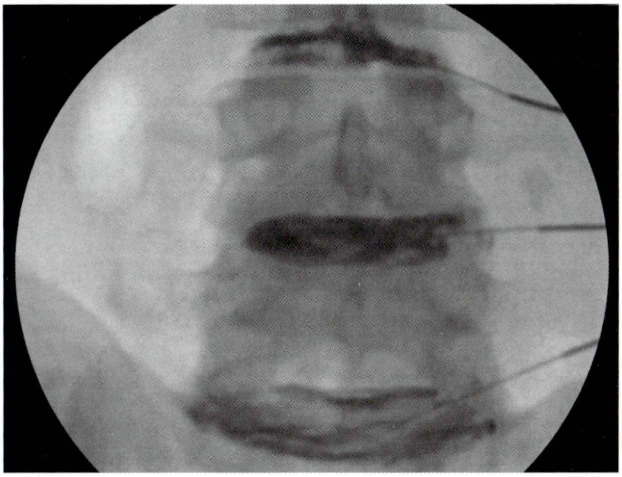

Fig. 16.2: Lumbar discogram with contrast noted in the discs at L3-4, L4-5 and L5-S1

possibility of infection. The patient received 1gm of cefazolin intra-venously prior to the procedure.

The C-arm was properly positioned toward the side noted above using an extradural approach. The soft tissues overlying the above levels were infiltrated with 4–6 cc of 1% lidocaine without epinephrine. An 18-gauge introducer needle was placed under fluoroscopic guidance to just posterior to each disc studied. A 22-gauge discography needle was then inserted into the center of the each lumbar disc. A mixture of 20 cc of omnipaque-240 and 200 mg of cefazolin was made sterilely. After confirmation of needle position on AP and lateral views, the contrast and antibiotic mixture was injected into each disc with a manometer. A nurse recorded the pressures, pain responses and nucleograms for each tested disc. Sham injections were also performed. Repeat confirmation for all levels' pain responses were done prior to cessation of the procedure.

Following the procedure, once the patient was confirmed to be stable, he was taken to the radiology suite for a post-discogram CT scan of the lumbar spine.

The patient tolerated the procedure well and without ill effects. He was provided our contact number and a small prescription for post-procedure discomfort. He was discharged with his wife at the end of the procedure.

Discography Results

Diagnosis: Internal disc disruption (IDD) syndrome
Levels tested: L3-4, L4-5, L5-S1
Approach: Extradural and infraneural, right

Discography Findings

- *L3-4*: No pain, opening pressure 15 PSI, nucleogram: cotton ball, max 100 PSI
- *L4-5*: Discordant pain, 2/10, opening pressure 15 PSI "location is too high," nucleogram: fissured, maximum pressure 100 PSI, pain at 50 PSI above opening pressure, no grimacing.
- *L5-S1*: Concordant pain, 8/10, opening pressure 10 PSI "you have found the spot", nucleogram: fissured with subligamentous protrusion, maximum PSI: 30 PSI, concordant pain at 10 PSI, facial grimacing.

Post-Discography Computed Tomography

- *L3-4*: cotton ball, contrast within the disc
- *L4-5*: Grade 1 tear, contrast within the disc
- *L5-S1*: Grade 3 tear, contrast within the disc and extravasating into epidural space.

Discography Impression

- *L3-4*: no pain, normal discogram.
- *L4-5*: discordant and mild pain, abnormal nucleogram.
- *L5-S1*: concordant pain at low pressure, abnormal nucleogram.

Impression: The above findings are consistent with IDD syndrome at L5-S1. All sham injections were negative. The pain findings were repeatable and consistent. The validity of the study was excellent.

DISCUSSION

Internal disc disruption syndrome (discogenic low back pain) is defined as pain resulting from a structurally and supportively incompetent lumbar intervertebral disc.[2] This often occurs as a result of injury, such as tears in the annulus fibrosis. The disc has been shown to contain pain-sensing fibers, reported first in 1975.[3] The outer annulus is innervated by the sinuvertebral nerves and gray rami communicantes.[4,5] These studies have also showed pain-producing chemicals such as substance P and calcitonin gene-related peptides and innervation in the outer annulus of damaged discs.[4-6] There are also both Ruffini and Golgi mechanoreceptors in the outer annulus fibrosis.[7] This has been demonstrated by pathologic staining of the disc.

Much of the current on chronic low back pain secondary to IDD is based on the theory of sensitization. The studies from Coppes suggest a neural "ingrowth" in individuals suffering from IDD.[4,5,8] Studies in rat and rabbit models have supported this theory.[9,10] The belief is that the torn disc may develop sprouting neural fibers that are pain sensing. These fibers may become hyper-excitable and cause a chronic pain syndrome. Studies of fetal discs and cadaveric discs have shown that the disc has innervation irrespective of disc degeneration, but that ingrowth may be a reason for sensitization.[11,12] Genetic factors may also play a role.[6]

The diagnosis of IDD is mostly clinical. Primarily axial low back pain with radiation to the buttocks and/or thigh, but not below the knee is common. This pain is normally provoked by sitting, standing, bending and twisting. Coughing or sneezing, and Valsalva may also provoke pain. Further support is made when MRI imaging demonstrates a disc with a high intensity zone (HIZ) on T2-weighted imaging in the posterior annulus.[13] Studies have shown a high correlation with concordant lower back pain with provocative lumbar discography and the presence of an HIZ.[13-18] Not all patients with an HIZ have pain, however.[15,18,19] Carragee showed a false positive rate of 25% in asymptomatic individuals.[20]

Lumbar provocative discography was declared the gold standard for the diagnosis of IDD syndrome by the North American Spine Society in 1988 and remains the diagnostic test for confirmation of discogenic pain.[21-23] It is a tool that can be utilized to confirm the diagnosis and, arguably, prevent unnecessary procedures performed for other causes of axial back pain (e.g. zygapophysial injections, sacroiliac joint injections).[2]

Internal disc disruption treatment and workup remains a topic of controversy.[24] The role of discography has been questioned since its inception in 1948.[24,25] A study from Holt in prisoners showed a high false positive rate of 36% with injection of noxious stimulus.[26] This was later refuted by Simmons due to the patient population, the use of an irritating contrast agent and technical approach.[27]

Several studies have since supported and refuted the utility and safety of lumbar discography. In the same year as the Holt paper, Wiley reported on the safety of the procedure showing relatively low complication rate.[28] Much controversy has existed on whether the procedure is accurate for in the assessment of disc pain as the nature of the procedure involves patient response. A study from Gruber et al. showed harmful effects of radiocontrast agents on nucleus cells in vitro.[29] Carragee et al. followed patients who had undergone provocative discography over 10 years and demonstrated an increased rate of degeneration and a higher incidence of far lateral disc herniations on the ipsilateral side as the disc entry point.[30] Carragee also showed a false positive rate of approximately 25% in low pressure lumbar discography.[31] Carragee also showed a high false positive rate of provocative discography in patients with chronic backache.[32] A study from Willems et al. did not show a substantial benefit in studying adjacent discs in patients who underwent fusion.[33]

Other studies support the use of discography in certain clinical situations. Berg et al. showed that discography has good utility in the surgical decision-making process.[34] Manchikanti et al. showed fair evidence for the use of discography in a retrospective analysis.[35] Manchikanti et al. also showed level II-2 evidence for the use of lumbar and cervical discography by reproduction of concordant pain via a "best evidence synthesis."[36] Resnick et al. purport utility in using discography to evaluate potential adjacent level disease in post-fusion patients and in abnormal discs for surgical consideration.[37]

The biggest risk associated with discography is infection due to the relatively poor vascular supply of the intervertebral disc as most of its nutrition occurs via diffusion in a relatively anerobic environment.[38] It is recommended to give preprocedure antibiotics such as cefazolin or clindamycin intravenously.[2] Sterile technique is a must and a thorough sterile prep is essential. While not a standard, we recommend a two-needle technique with an introduce needle through the skin and soft tissues and a spinal needle through this, which does not touch the skin. This allows the needle entering the disc to have minimal contact with anything but the disc itself.

The evaluation of the pain response to the studied disc is reported as "no pain," "discordant" (nontypical) or "concordant" (identical). Only concordant pain is considered positive. A numeric pain score may also be utilized and the patient's description of the pain documented to give more "objective" information. Facial grimacing is also useful as an indicator of the pain response.

Pressure recording with the production of pain is also utilized and important in the interpretation of the discogram. Opening pressure is defined as the pressure recorded on the manometer when contrast is first observed to enter the disc. The pressure at which pain is first observed is also recorded, as well as the pressure at the end of testing, or final pressure. The "Derby Criteria" are a well-described method of interpreting discography. The pain and pressure responses must show a concordant response of greater than 6/10 on a numeric pain scale at a pressure of less than 50 psi above the opening pressure and a negative control disc.[39] Also, the nucleogram must be abnormal, showing a grade 3 tear on the Dallas discogram scale (described below).

The nucleogram is also described in the report and lends credence to positive results. The Dallas discogram scale, described by Sachs et al. grades the disruption of the intervertebral disc as demonstrated by post-CT pictures on a scale of 0–3.[40] A "normal" nucleogram (Grade 0) is described as a cotton-ball appearance with contrast staying only in the disc. A Grade 1 tear extends into the inner third of the disc, Grade 2 to the middle third, and a Grade 3 to the outer third.[40] The post-discography CT scan also confirms that all injections are within the nucleus as annular injections are not reliable.

TREATMENT OPTIONS

The conservative treatment options for IDD often start with a physical therapy program with an emphasis on core strengthening. Proper lifting mechanics are emphasized and avoidance of aggravating factors, particularly sitting improperly and for extended periods of time should be avoided. The patient should be counseled to stop smoking as this may have deleterious effects on his pain, disc healing and overall health.[41,42] The patient should be counseled on the benign nature of the condition as "fear-avoidance" can significantly impact their willingness to exercise and glean quality of life.[43] Medications such as muscle relaxants, anti-inflammatories, antidepressants and narcotics may be considered but have questionable long-term benefits.[44-47]

Intradiscal procedures of varying types have been trialled. Chemonucleolysis with chymopapain, derived from papaya extract had been widely utilized and shown benefit in several studies,[48-50] but the company ceased its production in 2003. Serious complications including paraplegia and anaphylaxis have been reported.[51-55]

Intradiscal electrothermal annuloplasty (IDET) is a procedure where a catheter is placed into the disc and attached to a thermal generator. The catheter is then heated to approximately 90°C to cauterize the disc and destroy the pain fibers. It is also postulated to cause the disc tissue to harden.[56] The efficacy of IDET was called into question showing it helped approximately 50% of people attain about 50% reduction in their preprocedure pain.[57]

Biacuplasty is a procedure in which two radio- frequency probes are placed fluoroscopically in the left and right posterior disc. A radiofrequency current is then applied between the probes with a goal to heat the posterior annulus to 55–60°C. It has shown benefit in a selected population and has comparable results to IDET.[58-60]

While beyond the scope of this text, discography is often utilized in determining if a patient is a candidate for surgical discectomy and fusion. A serious conversation is needed with the patient prior to recommending this procedure, both by the surgeon and the discographer. The success rates for lumbar fusion for discogenic low back pain are reported to be between 50% and 70%.[61] One study showed no difference in outcome with surgery compared to psychological counseling.[62]

SUMMARY

The treatment of discogenic low back pain is challenging and research is currently being performed for disc-preserving, nonsurgical treatments. A serious discussion should be had with the patient regarding IDD and realistic goals of treatment explained. A multidisciplinary approach and conservative care should be maximized. If the patient's quality of life is significantly impaired and they are serious about pursuing surgical options for the pain, consideration of discography can be made. Counseling about the risks of the procedure including potential for harm to the disc should be made prior to the discogram. As with other procedures, proper patient selection is key and exclusion of psychiatric comorbidities should be made as this may potentially influence surgical outcomes, as well.[63-65]

REFERENCES

1. Porter SE, Hanley EN. The musculoskeletal effects of smoking. J Am Acad Orthop Surg. 2001;9(1):9-17.
2. Bogduk N. Spinal Diagnostic and Treatment Procedures: Practice Guidelines, 1st edition. San Francisco, CA: International Spine Intervention Society; 2004.
3. Shinohara H. [Lumbar disc lesion, with special reference to the histological significance of nerve endings of the lumbar discs]. Nihon Seikeigeka Gakkai Zasshi 1970;44(8):553-70.
4. Coppes MH, Marani E, Thomeer RT, et al. Innervation of annulus fibrosis in low back pain. Lancet. 1990;336(8708):189-90.
5. Coppes MH, Marani E, Thomeer RT, et al. Innervation of "painful" lumbar discs. Spine. 1997;22(20):2342-9.
6. Kepler CK, Ponnappan RK, Tannoury CA, et al. The molecular basis of intervertebral disc degeneration. Spine J. 2013;13(3):318-30.
7. Dimitroulias A, Tsonidis C, Natsis K, et al. An immunohistochemical study of mechanoreceptors in lumbar spine intervertebral discs. J Clin Neurosci. 2010;17(6):742-5.
8. Takahashi K, Aoki Y, Ohtori S. Resolving discogenic pain. Eur Spine J. 2008;17 Suppl 4:428-31.
9. Inoue G, Ohtori S, Aoki Y, et al. Exposure of the nucleus pulposus to the outside of the anulus fibrosus induces nerve injury and regeneration of the afferent fibers innervating the lumbar intervertebral discs in rats. Spine. 2006;31(13):1433-8.
10. Aoki Y, Akeda K, An H, et al. Nerve fiber ingrowth into scar tissue formed following nucleus pulposus extrusion in the rabbit anular-puncture disc degeneration model: effects of depth of puncture. Spine. 2006;31(21):E774-80.
11. Edgar MA. The nerve supply of the lumbar intervertebral disc. J Bone Joint Surg Br. 2007;89(9):1135-9.
12. Peng B, Wu W, Hou S, et al. The pathogenesis of discogenic low back pain. J Bone Joint Surg Br. 2005;87(1):62-7.
13. Aprill C, Bogduk N. High-intensity zone: a diagnostic sign of painful lumbar disc on magnetic resonance imaging. Br J Radiol. 1992;65(773):361-9.
14. Peng B, Hou S, Wu W, et al. The pathogenesis and clinical significance of a high-intensity zone (HIZ) of lumbar intervertebral disc on MR imaging in the patient with discogenic low back pain. Eur Spine J. . 2006;15:583-7.
15. Lam KS, Carlin D, Mulholland RC. Lumbar disc high-intensity zone: the value and significance of provocative discography in the determination of the discogenic pain source. Eur Spine J. 2000;9:36-41.
16. Wang ZX, Hu YG, Chen XM. [Significance of the high-intensity zone located in the posterior annulus fibrosus for diagnosing discogenic low back pain]. Zhonghua Yi Xue Za Zhi. 2008;88(35):2478-81.

17. Wang HD, Hou SX, Wang XN, et al. [Correlation between high intensity zone on MRI and positive pain response on lumbar discography in the diagnosis of discogenic low back pain]. Zhonghua Wai Ke Za Zhi. 2008;46(13):973-6.
18. Kang CH, Kim YH, Lee SH, et al. Can magnetic resonance imaging accurately predict concordant pain provocation during provocative disc injection? Skeletal Radiol. 2009;38(9):877-85.
19. Carragee EJ, Barcohana B, Alamin T, et al. Prospective controlled study of the development of lower back pain in previously asymptomatic subjects undergoing experimental discography. Spine. 2004;29(10):1112-7.
20. Carragee EJ, Paragioudakis SJ, Khurana S. 2000 Volvo Award winner in clinical studies: Lumbar high-intensity zone and discography in subjects without low back problems. Spine. 2000;25(23):2987-92.
21. Guyer RD, Ohnmeiss DD. Lumbar discography. Position statement from the North American Spine Society Diagnostic and Therapeutic Committee. Spine. 1995;20(18):2048-59.
22. Maus TP, Aprill CN. Lumbar diskogenic pain, provocation diskography, and imaging correlates. Radiol Clin North Am. 2012;50(4):681-704.
23. Guyer RD, Ohnmeiss DD, Nass. Lumbar discography. Spine J. 2003;3(3 Suppl):11S-27S.
24. Carragee EJ, Lincoln T, Parmar VS, et al. A gold standard evaluation of the "discogenic pain" diagnosis as determined by provocative discography. Spine. 2006;31(18):2115-23.
25. Lindblom K. Diagnostic puncture of intervertebral disks in sciatica. Acta Orthop Scand. 1948;17(3-4):231-9.
26. Holt EP. The question of lumbar discography. J Bone Joint Surg Am. 1968;50(4):720-6.
27. Simmons JW, Aprill CN, Dwyer AP, et al. A reassessment of Holt's data on: "The question of lumbar discography". Clin Orthop Relat Res. 1988;(237):120-4.
28. Wiley JJ, Macnab I, Wortzman G. Lumbar discography and its clinical applications. Can J Surg. 1968;11(3):280-9.
29. Gruber HE, Rhyne AL, Hansen KJ, et al. Deleterious effects of discography radiocontrast solution on human annulus cell in vitro: changes in cell viability, proliferation, and apoptosis in exposed cells. Spine J. 2012;12:329-35.
30. Carragee EJ, Don AS, Hurwitz EL, et al. 2009 ISSLS Prize Winner: Does discography cause accelerated progression of degeneration changes in the lumbar disc: a ten-year matched cohort study. Spine. 2009;34(21):2338-45.
31. Carragee EJ, Alamin TF, Carragee JM. Low-pressure positive Discography in subjects asymptomatic of significant low back pain illness. Spine. 2006;31(5):505-9.
32. Carragee EJ, Alamin TF, Miller J, et al. Provocative discography in volunteer subjects with mild persistent low back pain. Spine J. 2002;2(1):25-34.
33. Willems PC, Elmans L, Anderson PG, et al. Provocative discography and lumbar fusion: is preoperative assessment of adjacent discs useful? Spine. 2007;32(10):1094-9; discussion 1100.
34. Berg S, Isberg B, Josephson A, et al. The impact of discography on the surgical decision in patients with chronic low back pain. Spine J. 2012;12(4):283-91.
35. Manchikanti L, Datta S, Derby R, et al. A critical review of the American Pain Society clinical practice guidelines for interventional techniques: part 1. Diagnostic interventions. Pain Physician. 2010;13(3):E141-74.

36. Manchikanti L, Boswell MV, Singh V, et al. Comprehensive review of neurophysiologic basis and diagnostic interventions in managing chronic spinal pain. Pain Physician. 2009;12(4):E71-120.
37. Resnick DK, Choudhri TF, Dailey AT, et al. Guidelines for the performance of fusion procedures for degenerative disease of the lumbar spine. Part 6: magnetic resonance imaging and discography for patient selection for lumbar fusion. J Neurosurg Spine. 2005;2(6):662-9.
38. Holm S, Maroudas A, Urban JP, et al. Nutrition of the intervertebral disc: solute transport and metabolism. Connect Tissue Res. 1981;8(2):101-19.
39. Derby R, Lee SH, Kim BJ, et al. Pressure-controlled lumbar discography in volunteers without low back symptoms. Pain Med. 2005;6(3):213-21.
40. Sachs BL, Vanharanta H, Spivey MA, et al. Dallas discogram description. A new classification of CT/discography in low-back disorders. Spine. 1987;12(3): 287-94.
41. Palmer KT, Syddall H, Cooper C, et al. Smoking and musculoskeletal disorders: findings from a British national survey. Ann Rheum Dis. 2003;62(1):33-6.
42. Alkherayf F, Agbi C. Cigarette smoking and chronic low back pain in the adult population. Clin Invest Med. 2009;32(5):E360-7.
43. Rainville J, Smeets RJ, Bendix T, et al. Fear-avoidance beliefs and pain avoidance in low back pain--translating research into clinical practice. Spine J. 2011;11(9):895-903.
44. Wielage R, Bansal M, Wilson K, et al. The Cost-Effectiveness of Duloxetine in Chronic Low Back Pain: a Quebec Societal Perspective. Spine. 2012.
45. Anastassopoulos KP, Chow W, Tapia CI, et al. Economic study on the impact of side effects in patients taking oxycodone controlled-release for noncancer pain. J Manag Care Pharm. 2012;18(8):615-26.
46. Casazza BA. Diagnosis and treatment of acute low back pain. Am Fam Physician. 2012;85(4):343-50.
47. Martell BA, O'Connor PG, Kerns RD, et al. Systematic review: opioid treatment for chronic back pain: prevalence, efficacy, and association with addiction. Ann Intern Med. 2007;146(2):116-27.
48. Wittenberg RH, Oppel S, Rubenthaler FA, et al. Five-year results from chemonucleolysis with chymopapain or collagenase: a prospective randomized study. Spine. 2001;26(17):1835-41.
49. Simmons JW, Nordby EJ, Hadjipavlou AG. Chemonucleolysis: the state of the art. Eur Spine J. 2001;10(3):192-202.
50. Kim YS, Chin DK, Yoon DH, et al. Predictors of successful outcome for lumbar chemonucleolysis: analysis of 3000 cases during the past 14 years. Neurosurgery. 2002;51(5 Suppl):S123-8.
51. Benoist M, Bex C, Lassale B, et al. [Neurological complications of chemonucleolysis with chymopapain. Apropos of a case]. Rev Rhum Mal Osteoart. 1987;54(10):651-4.
52. Boccanera L, Laus M. Chemonucleolysis: advantages and disadvantages. Chir Organi Mov. 1990;75(1):25-32.
53. Haag P, Munkel K, Meinck HM. [Late myelopathy after chemonucleolysis. Case report and review of the literature]. Nervenarzt. 1999;70(10):920-3.
54. Dabezies EJ, Langford K, Morris J, et al. Safety and efficacy of chymopapain (Discase) in the treatment of sciatica due to a herniated nucleus pulposus. Results of a randomized, double-blind study. Spine. 1988;13(5):561-5.

55. Kitchel SH, Brown MD. Complications of chemonucleolysis. Clin Orthop Relat Res. 1992;(284):63-74.
56. Saal JA, Saal JS. Intradiscal electrothermal treatment for chronic discogenic low back pain: prospective outcome study with a minimum 2-year follow-up. Spine. 2002;27(9):966-73.
57. Pauza KJ, Howell S, Dreyfuss P, et al. A randomized, placebo-controlled trial of intradiscal electrothermal therapy for the treatment of discogenic low back pain. Spine J. 2004;4(1):27-35.
58. Kapural L, Vrooman B, Sarwar S, et al. A randomized, placebo-controlled trial of transdiscal radiofrequency, biacuplasty for treatment of discogenic lower back pain. Pain Med. 2013;14(3):362-73.
59. Kapural L, Ng A, Dalton J, et al. Intervertebral disc biacuplasty for the treatment of lumbar discogenic pain: results of a six-month follow-up. Pain Med. 2008;9(1):60-7.
60. Karaman H, Tufek A, Kavak GO, et al. 6-month results of TransDiscal Biacuplasty on patients with discogenic low back pain: preliminary findings. Int J Med Sci. 2010;8(1):1-8.
61. Guyer RD, McAfee PC, Banco RJ, et al. Prospective, randomized, multicenter Food and Drug Administration investigational device exemption study of lumbar total disc replacement with the CHARITE artificial disc versus lumbar fusion: five-year follow-up. Spine J. 2009;9:374-86.
62. Brox JI, Sorensen R, Friis A, et al. Randomized clinical trial of lumbar instrumented fusion and cognitive intervention and exercises in patients with chronic low back pain and disc degeneration. Spine. 2003;28:1913-21.
63. Carragee EJ. Psychological screening in the surgical treatment of lumbar disc herniation. Clin J Pain. 2001;17(3):215-9.
64. Carragee EJ. Psychological and functional profiles in select subjects with low back pain. Spine J. 2001;1(3):198-204.
65. Derby R, Lettice JJ, Kula TA, et al. Single-level lumbar fusion in chronic discogenic low-back pain: psychological and emotional status as a predictor of outcome measured using the 36-item Short Form. J Neurosurg Spine. 2005;3(4):255-61.

17

Thoracic Facet Pain

Michael J Mehnert, Jesse A Sally, Gary P Chimes

CHIEF COMPLAINT

The patient complains of persistent "mid-back pain".

HISTORY OF PRESENT ILLNESS

A 54-year-old man with no significant past medical history presents to the office with the above complaint. He reports that for the past 18 months he has had increasing pain in the mid-back area between the shoulder blades, (Fig. 17.1) and does not recall any specific injury. He has had episodes of his "back going out" a few times a year for as long as he can remember, and believes he has "disc problems" in his mid- and lower spine. He complains of an aching and burning pain "with tingling right over that spot" that occurs toward the end of the day, in particular when he is on his feet. The pain is worse with standing and walking and much better with sitting. Sometimes the area is stiff and sore when he wakes up. Initially he was getting by with regular use of anti-inflammatories and muscle relaxants, but over the past 2 months his pain has increased to a 7–8 out of 10 and does not respond to medications. He has tried physical therapy and exercise, and had to stop walking on a treadmill for exercise due to increasing pain, but he can tolerate limited use of a recumbent bike. Heating modalities are helpful but have given less relief recently. He reports that when his symptoms become more severe such as when standing at work, he finds that bending forward to stretch decreases his pain.

He has no history of shingles or constitutional symptoms. He denies night time pain. The pain does not radiate along the ribcage or into the low back and he denies numbness, tingling or weakness in the lower limbs.

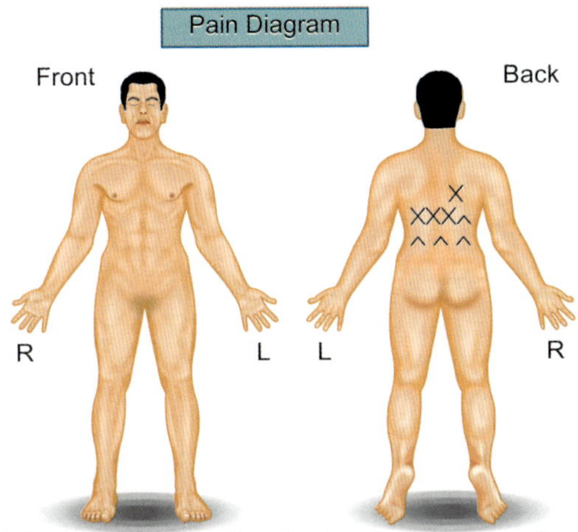

Using the symbols below, the location and type of pain sensations are marked on the diagrams. All the affected areas are included.

TYPE OF SENSATIONS

Aching	^ ^ ^ ^ ^ ^
Burning	X X X X X X
Sharp or stabbing	//////////
Pins and needles	0 0 0 0 0 0
Numbness	II II II II II II

Fig. 17.1: Pain diagram

PAST MEDICAL HISTORY

Hypertension, reflux disease

PAST SURGICAL HISTORY

Left shoulder rotator cuff repair

REVIEW OF SYSTEMS

As per history of present illness and also remark-able for fatigue, weight gain and seasonal allergies.

FAMILY HISTORY

None significant

SOCIAL HISTORY

He reports no current tobacco use (quit smoking 11 years ago) and no illicit drug use. He consumes one to two beers per day. He works as an electrical engineer.

CURRENT MEDICATIONS

Hydrochlorothiazide. Also cyclobenzaprine and ibuprofen as needed.

ALLERGIES

Sulfa medications

PHYSICAL EXAMINATION

- *Height*: 5'11"
- *Weight*: 224 lbs
- *BMI*: 31.2
- *Pulse*: 84/minute
- *BP*: 128/82 mm Hg
- *Respirations*: 9/minute

This is an alert, awake and cooperative male. Nutrition and hygiene are well-maintained. He is overweight and he appears uncomfortable during the interview, changing position occasionally.

He ambulates with a normal gait and station and can do heel-and-toe walking.

Coordination is intact in the upper and lower limbs.

Thoracolumbar spine exam demonstrates normal overlying skin without erythema, edema, or surgical scar. No zoster skin lesions are appreciated.

Range of motion is full with reproducible pain at end range extension. Forward flexion is full and painless. Oblique extension is painful bilaterally, though more so on the right. Prolonged standing in spinal extension provokes an increase in axial pain between the shoulder blades without complaints of radiating or claudicating pain. The spinous processes are nontender. Focal tenderness is noted along the right greater than left thoracic paraspinals and the facet joints, approximating the T6-T8 levels. No palpable muscle spasm is appreciated; trigger points are not identified. Scapulohumeral motion is normal without winging.

Neurological exam demonstrates 5/5 strength in the upper and lower limbs in all key myotomes tested. Sensory testing to light touch and pinprick is normal in the upper and lower limbs in all key dermatomes tested. Sensory testing of thoracic dermatomes demonstrated normal sensation as well to light touch. Reflexes are 2+ and symmetric in the upper and lower limbs at the biceps, triceps, brachioradialis, patella and the Achilles.

Long tract signs are absent bilaterally.

Dural tension signs are negative in the lower limbs.

IMAGING

X-Rays

Anteroposterior, lateral, flexion and extension views of the lumbar spine were normal. Disc height was well-maintained throughout except at L5-S1 where loss of disc-space height is noted with some endplate changes and facet arthropathy. Lumbar lordosis is normal and no instability is noted on flexion or extension.

Anteroposterior and lateral views of the thoracic spine were obtained. No evidence of fracture is appreciated and no scoliosis is identified. Spur formation is noted anteriorly at several levels, with loss of disc height at T6-T7 and T7-T8.

Magnetic Resonance Imaging

Magnetic resonance imaging of the thoracic spine without contrast demonstrates disc desiccation at T6-T7 and T7-T8. Loss of disc height is appreciated at these same two levels. Facet arthropathy is noted at T6-T7 as well. Spinal cord signal is normal. No nerve root compression or cord compression is identified.

DIAGNOSIS

Thoracic zygapophysial joint pain (thoracic facet syndrome)—likely involving the right greater than left T6-T7 and T7-T8 zygapophysial joints. The patient describes axial pain between the shoulder blades in the region of the thoracic zygapophysial joints. Symptoms are reportedly and demonstrably worse with extension-biased activities and maneuvers and extension-rotation movements. A lack of radicular pain and neuropathic symptoms is also consistent with this diagnosis.

DIFFERENTIAL DIAGNOSIS

For this patient, the differential diagnosis would also include other causes of axial spine pain, such as soft-tissue pathology (myofascial pain, muscle sprain) though this would be less likely given an absence of trigger points or appreciable muscle spasm on exam. This patient could also be symptomatic from thoracic degenerative disc disease, but reproduction of pain with "loading" of the facet joints with extension and oblique extension along with tenderness to palpation is more consistent with zygapophysial joint pain or other posterior element pathology. Improvement in pain with sitting and flexion-biased stretches would also point toward pain from the posterior zygapophysial joints and would make discogenic pain less likely as well.[1] The patient's MRI results and lack of sensory deficits and neuropathic pain symptoms would make a thoracic radiculopathy or zoster infection much less likely.

Thoracic Zygapophysial Joint Pain

Diagnosis and treatment of thoracic zygapophysial joint pain has evolved as a clinical entity analogous to cervical and lumbar zygapophysial joint pain.[2,3] The thoracic zygapophysial joints are true synovial-lined joints.[4,5] Sprains and contusions of the zygapophysial joints in the thoracic spinal regions, as well as osteoarthritis, have been postulated as causes of axial thoracic spine pain mediated by the zygapophysial joints.[6] Pain patterns attributable to the thoracic zygapophysial joints when they are noxiously stimulated to become "pain generators" have been described in the literature[7,8] (Figs 17.2A and B). In the lumbar spine, imaging studies have not been shown to be useful indicators of facet joint pain,[9] though there is a role in imaging to rule-out other causes of pain. Physical exam is also not sufficient to accurately diagnose facet-mediated pain.[10]

TREATMENT OPTIONS

As with other conditions that can cause axial spine pain, initial treatment should be conservative and include medication management, physical therapy, modalities and potentially spinal manipulation. A regular home exercise program as well as activity modification should be incorporated. Weight loss should be encouraged. Anti-inflammatory medications may be preferred; opioid usage should be avoided if possible.

Interventional Options

Dogmatic interventional treatment approaches for thoracic zygapophysial joint pain are analogous to those available for cervical and lumbar zygapophysial joint pain and include corticosteroid/anesthetic injections intra-articularly, anesthetic blockade of the corresponding medial branches and sensory innervation, as well as standard radiofrequency neurotomy of the same medial branches. Pulsed radiofrequency of the thoracic medial branches lacks sufficient evidence at this time, and other denervation techniques (chemodenervation) have been described but are less commonly employed.[11]

Sensory innervation to the thoracic zygapophysial joints is analogous to the lumbar zygapophysial joints both in terms of responsible neural

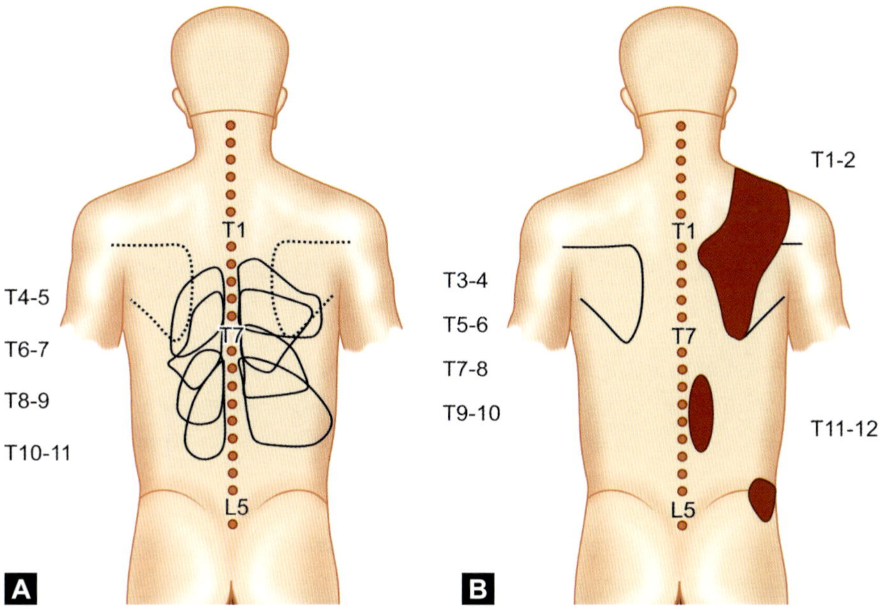

Figs 17.2A and B: Maps of referred pain patterns in normal volunteers elicited by noxious stimulation of the thoracic zygapophysial joints at the segments indicated
Source: (A) Dreyfuss et al.; (B) Fukui et al.

structures and also the numbering of the individual zygapophysial joints and their corresponding nerve roots and medial branches.[12-14] Two medial branch nerves originating from two different dorsal rami innervate each joint. Care must be taken to clearly identify the target joint (often identified as two levels with a hyphen, i.e. the T3-T4 zygapophysial joint) and the corresponding medial branches (often identified with a comma, i.e. the T2, T3 medial branches). Additionally, the medial branches are often accessed at a vertebral transverse process one level below the actual name of the originating nerve root. For example, the T3-T4 zygapophysial joint can be anesthetized by injecting anesthetic with a needle upon the T2 medial branch as it crosses the transverse process of the T3 vertebral body and upon the T3 medial branch as it crosses the transverse process of the T4 vertebral body.[2,14,15]

There may be a role for intra-articular corticosteroid injections, particularly for osteoarthritic joints.[16,17] However, the role of a diagnostic joint injection is well-established.[16-19] The thoracic articulating joints are oriented in a near-coronal plane and thus access from a direct posterior needle approach is often prohibited by the overlying vertebral lamina.[20] Similarly the unique anatomy of the thoracic spine with the pulmonary structures in close proximity precludes needle access to the thoracic facet joints from a lateral approach.[6] Nonetheless, an intra-articular approach accessing the inferior aspect of a thoracic facet joint has been described.[6,21]

Medial branch blocks are also a diagnostic intervention, utilized to determine if a given zygapophysial joint can be considered the source of a patient's pain. Comparative medial branch blocks are employed for diagnostic purposes, in accordance with a validated model for cervical zygapophysial joint pain.[22-24] Data exclusive to thoracic zygapophysial joint pain are, by comparison to the cervical literature, limited.[25] Anesthetic blocks on at least two separate occasions should be performed; however, the exact criteria for positive comparative blocks with two different local anesthetics can be left up to the physician.[2] Some authors advocate complete abolition of pain with diagnostic blockade[2] where others have suggested a threshold of 80% pain relief.[26] It has been demonstrated that a single-block paradigm for thoracic medial branches can have a false positive rate of 58%.[25]

The location of the potential target thoracic medial branches (Figs 17.3 and 17.4) has also been described via cadaver analysis[14,15] in a manner similar to that for the cervical medial branches.[27]

An initial technique for thoracic medial branch blocks (and subsequent percutaneous neurotomy) was initially described by Stolker et al.[28] Anatomical studies of the location of the thoracic medial branches by Chua[14] conclude that this technique is inaccurate.[2]

Localization of a target painful thoracic zygapophysial joint with medial branch blocks should be done only with the expectation that a patient would be willing to move on to a medial branch neurotomy procedure.[2] Thoracic zygapophysial joint pain *must* be confirmed with prior diagnostic medial branch blocks before advancing to a neurotomy procedure for pain control.

Thoracic medial branch radiofrequency neurotomy potentially offers the advantage of longer-term pain relief from a problematic thoracic zygapophysial joint. Over 1 year of pain relief can be expected.[29-31]

The location of the target thoracic medial branches is appreciably different from that in the cervical and lumbar spine.[2,14] Furthermore the thoracic medial branches demonstrate significant variability (Figs 17.3 and 17.4) in their location throughout the thoracic levels.[14,26] Nonetheless, the equipment, sensory and motor stimulation, and the radiofrequency lesioning protocol are otherwise similar to that utilized in the lumbar spine.[2,26]

The above procedures are indicated for patients who, as a general rule, have failed to improve with more conservative measures. A reasonable suspicion of pain mediated by the thoracic zygapophysial joints should exist, and a target joint for anesthetic blockade or injection of corticosteroid is often chosen based on clinical exam findings and reported pain patterns.[18] Fluoroscopic guidance is necessary for accuracy, and the patient should keep a written pain diary to assess their level of response and minimize recall bias.[2,32,33]

Contraindications include active infection, coagulopathy/bleeding diathesis, pregnancy or allergy to a given injectate.[2]

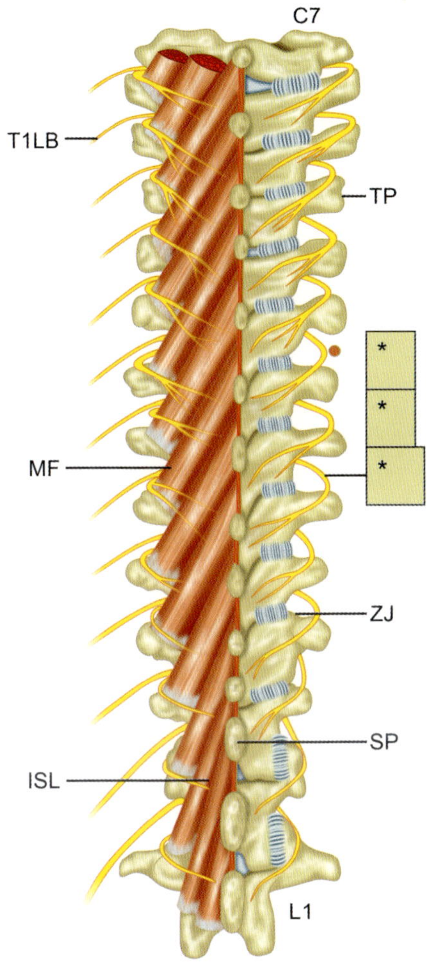

Fig. 17.3: A sketch of the thoracic medial branches from Chua[1]. Nerves with an atypical course are marked with an asterisk (*)

Plan/Treatment Course

Given the failure to achieve adequate pain relief with medications, physical therapy and activity modification, a decision was made to move forward with right-sided T6-T7 and T7-T8 intra-articular zygapophysial joint injections. Pain relief of 90% was reported, albeit temporarily. Sub-sequently, an injection procedure to anesthetize the medial branches that innervate the right-sided T6-T7 and T7-T8 zygapophysial joints was performed. Again significant, concordant pain-relief was obtained without complication. Ultimately, a decision was made to proceed with a radiofrequency neurotomy procedure to denervate the right T6-T7 and T7-T8 thoracic zygapophysial joints for better pain control.

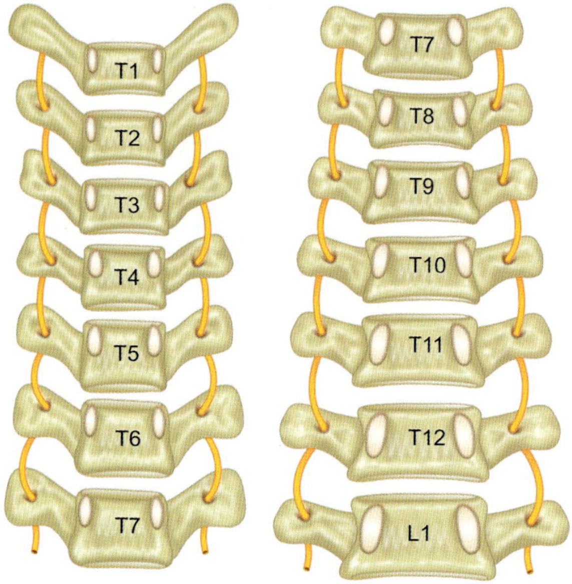

Fig. 17.4: A composite sketch of a radiograph of cada- veric thoracic spines in which the medial branches of the thoracic dorsal rami were marked with wires, in order to depict their relationship to the transverse processes. From Chua[1]. Note how at middle thoracic levels, the nerves are suspended in the intratransverse space, whereas at other levels they cross, and lie on, the transverse processes

Tricks and Tips

- During a neurotomy procedure relatively light sedation should be used so that the patient can be questioned for the perception of radiating or radicular pain during sensory stimulation and for the perception of nonmultifidus muscle contraction during motor stimulation. Similarly, narcotic medications or intravenous opioids should be administered after the stimulation portion of the neurotomy proce- dure.
- The operator should bear in mind that even light sedation and anxiolytics can potentially impact the patient's reporting of their response to a diagnostic injection.
- For intra-articular injections, expected volumes are often quite small (~1 mL including contrast media) and higher concentrations of cortico-steroid preparations to keep volumes lower may be useful.
- The level to be injected and accessed with a needle will need to be identified by counting the ribs to the target level (being careful that a cervical rib does not exist).
- Anatomic variability with regard to location of the traversing medial branches over a given thoracic spinous process can be significant; refer to the above anatomic locations when proceeding with neural blockade or neurotomy.[14,15]

Procedure Note—Thoracic Intra-articular Zygapophysial Joint Injection

Procedure

Thoracic facet joint injection (intra-articular injection) with fluoroscopic guidance

Indications

Please refer to prior office notes for details. The patient is being treated for a diagnosis of thoracic pain and thoracic facet syndrome. The patient has failed to respond to conservative measures including physiotherapy, medications, and activity modification. A decision was made to proceed with fluoroscopically-guided thoracic facet joint injections for diagnostic and possibly therapeutic purposes.

The patient was informed of the risks and benefits of the procedure, as well as alternative treatments. The risks include, but are not limited to, death, paralysis, allergic reaction, syncope, arrhythmia, cardiac or respiratory arrest, spinal cord injury, worse pain, scar formation, bleeding, epidural hematoma and infection. All questions were answered prior to proceeding. The patient expressed understanding and gave informed written consent.

Preoperative Diagnosis

Thoracic facet pain, thoracic facet syndrome

Postoperative Diagnosis

Same

Procedure Performed

- Thoracic intra-articular facet joint injection to the right T6-T7 and T7-T8 facet joints
- Fluoroscopic guidance/localization.

The patient was taken into the fluoroscopy suite and was placed prone on the procedure table. The patient was prepped and draped in a sterile fashion. All vital signs were monitored prior to, during, and after the procedure. Oxygen saturation was also monitored and noted to be greater than or equal to 94% throughout the procedure. Cardiac monitoring revealed normal sinus rhythm.

The C-arm was positioned so that the region overlying the right T6-T7 and T7-T8 zygapophysial joints was visualized. The soft tissues overlying these structures were infiltrated with 1% lidocaine without epinephrine and buffered with sodium bicarbonate for local anesthesia. Then, under

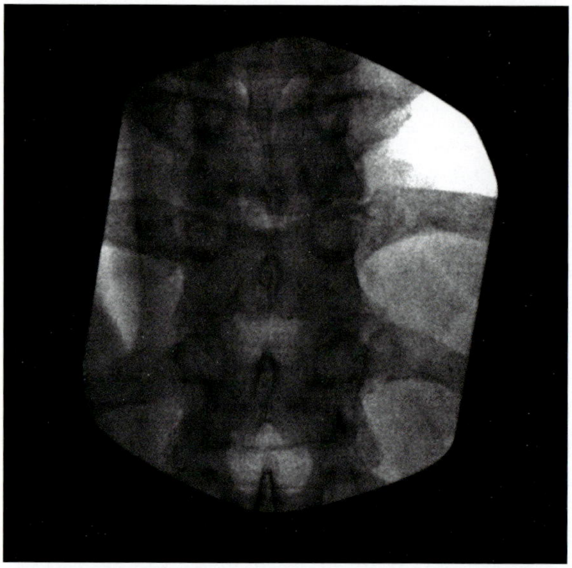

Fig. 17.5: A decline view of the needle approaching the target right thoracic facet joint

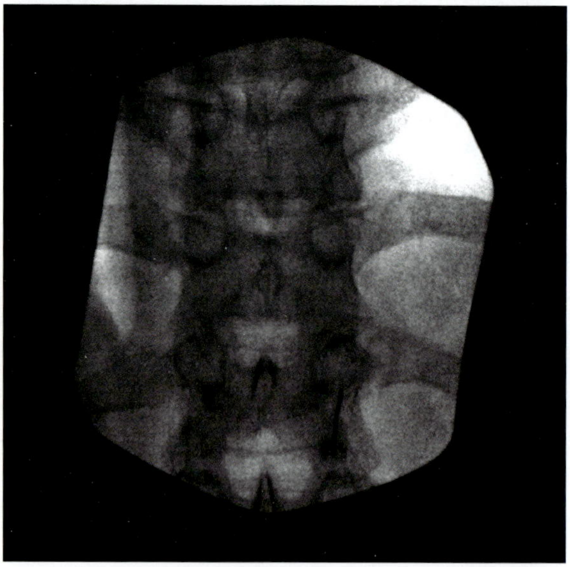

Fig. 17.6: An AP view of the needle approaching the target joint; note that the needle is advanced towards the joint from an inferior to superior approach

intermittent fluoroscopic guidance, a 25-gauge spinal needle was inserted into the inferior aspect of each of the above mentioned zygapophysial joints (Figs 17.5 and 17.6). Multiplanar fluoroscopic imaging was obtained to verify correct needle positioning (Figs 17.7 and 17.8).

After aspiration was attempted and was negative for return of blood or other fluid, a small amount of nonionic contrast was injected and flow of

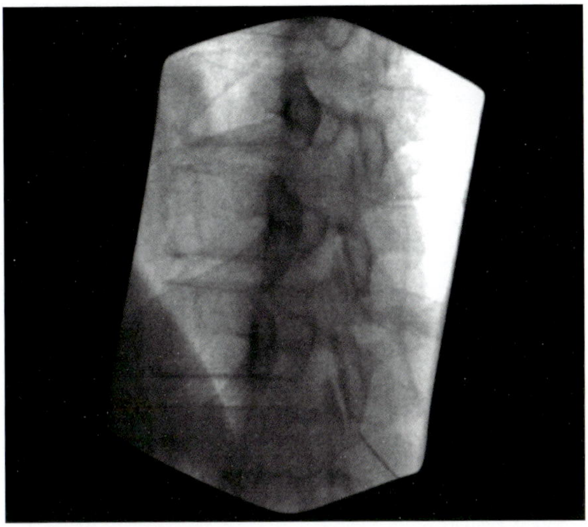

Fig. 17.7: A lateral view of the target joint with the needle approaching the target facet joint

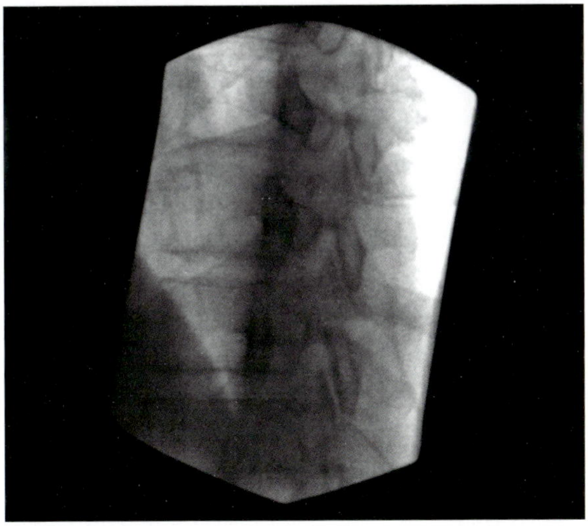

Fig. 17.8: A lateral view of the target joint with the needle approaching the joint; note that compared to the previous image the needle bevel was rotated to better access the intra-articular space

contrast was noted at each level (Figs 17.9 to 17.11), with care given to assess for vascular flow. Radiographs were obtained for documentation purposes. The injectate consisting of steroid and lidocaine was administered into each joint.

The needles were then withdrawn and hemostasis was achieved.

The patient tolerated the procedure well and was discharged after an appropriate period of observation. Postprocedure instructions were given and the patient was advised to call with any questions or concerns.

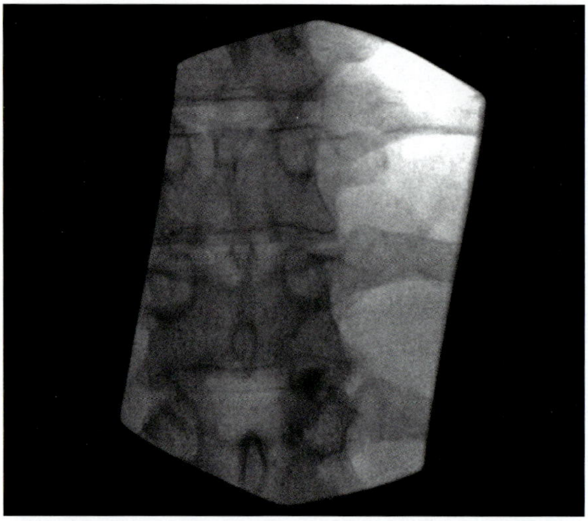

Fig. 17.9: A lateral view of the target joint with the needle in place and contrast filling the intra-articular space

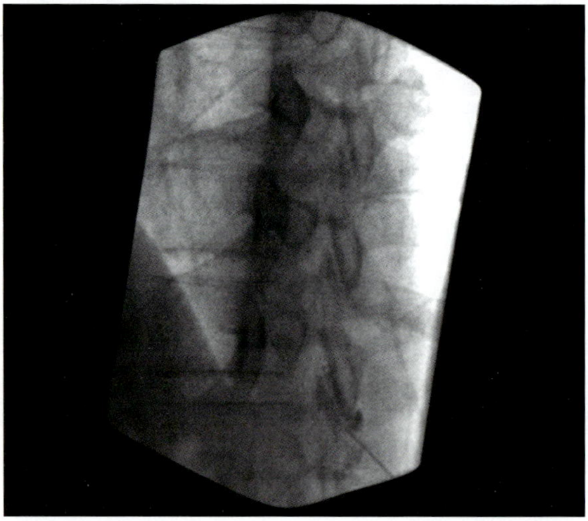

Fig. 17.10: An AP view of contrast in the target thoracic facet joint

The patient is to follow-up with the physician as noted above within 1–2 weeks.

The patient was also given a pain diary and was instructed to note the pain level and activities at the time of entering the data for the day of the procedure. The patient will bring this data to the follow-up appointment for diagnostic purposes.

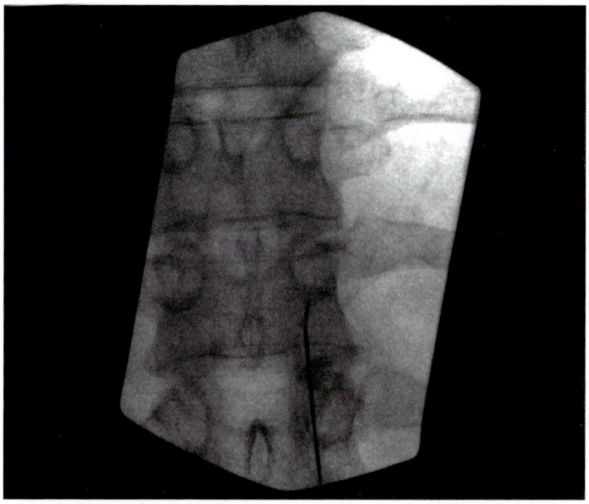

Fig. 17.11: The procedure being repeated to access a second joint superior to the previously injected facet joint

Procedure Note—Thoracic Medial Branch Block

Procedure

Thoracic medial branch block (zygapophysial joint nerve block) with fluoroscopic guidance.

Indications

Please refer to prior office notes for details. The patient is being treated for a diagnosis of thoracic pain and thoracic facet syndrome. The patient has failed to respond to conservative measures including physiotherapy, medications, and activity modification. A decision was made to proceed with fluoroscopically-guided thoracic medial branch blocks for diagnostic purposes.

The patient was informed of the risks and benefits of the procedure, as well as alternative treatments. The risks include, but are not limited to death, paralysis, allergic reaction, syncope, arrhythmia, cardiac or respiratory arrest, spinal cord injury, worse pain, scar formation, bleeding, epidural hematoma and infection. All questions were answered prior to proceeding. The patient expressed understanding and gave informed written consent.

Preoperative Diagnosis

Thoracic facet pain, thoracic facet syndrome

Postoperative Diagnosis

Same

Procedure Performed

- Thoracic medial branch blocks to the right T5, T6 and T7 nerves to anesthetize the right T6-T7 and T7-T8 thoracic facet joints
- Fluoroscopic guidance/localization.

The patient was taken into the fluoroscopy suite and was placed prone on the procedure table. The patient was prepped and draped in a sterile fashion. All vital signs were monitored prior to, during, and after the procedure. Oxygen saturation was also monitored and noted to be greater than or equal to 94% throughout the procedure. Cardiac monitoring revealed normal sinus rhythm.

The C-arm was positioned so that the T6, T7 and T8 vertebrae were identified. The soft tissues overlying these structures were anesthetized with 1% lidocaine without epinephrine and buffered with sodium bicarbonate as a local anesthetic.

At the T6 vertebrae, a 25-gauge spinal needle was advanced down via an oblique approach to the site of the traversing medial branch on the transverse process of the vertebra on the right side. This corresponds to the right T5 medial branch nerve. Needle positioning was done under intermittent fluoroscopic guidance.

At the T7 vertebrae, a 25-gauge spinal needle was advanced down via an oblique approach to the site of the traversing medial branch on the transverse process of the vertebra on the right side. This corresponds to the right T6 medial branch nerve. Needle positioning was done under intermittent fluoroscopic guidance (Fig. 17.12).

At the T8 vertebrae, a 25-gauge spinal needle was advanced down via an oblique approach to the site of the traversing medial branch on the transverse process of the vertebra on the right side. This corresponds to the right T7 medial branch nerve. Needle positioning was done under intermittent fluoroscopic guidance.

An AP view was obtained to verify correct needle positioning. After aspiration was attempted and was negative for return of blood or other fluid, a small amount of nonionic contrast was injected and flow of contrast was noted at each level, with care given to assess for vascular flow. Radiographs were obtained for documentation purposes. Next, the selected preservative-free local anesthetic was administered at each level.

The needles were then withdrawn and hemostasis was achieved.

The patient tolerated the procedure well and was discharged after an appropriate period of observation. Postprocedure instructions were given

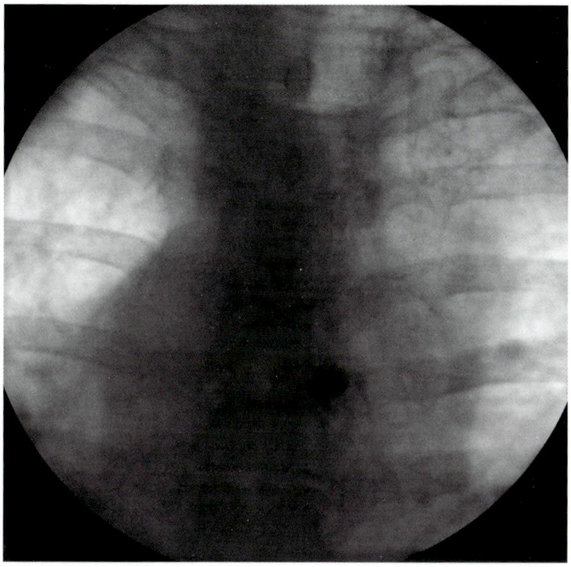

Fig. 17.12: Example of an AP view of the needle in place at the site of the traversing medial branch for a different patient

and the patient was advised to call with any questions or concerns. The patient is to follow-up with the physician as noted above within 1–2 weeks.

The patient was also given a pain diary and was instructed to note the pain level and activities at the time of entering the data for the day of the procedure. The patient will bring this data to the follow-up appointment for diagnostic purposes.

Procedure Note—Radiofrequency Neurotomy of Thoracic Medial Branches

Procedure

Radiofrequency neurotomy of the thoracic medial branches (zygapophysial joint nerve ablation) with fluoroscopic guidance.

Indications

Please refer to prior office notes for details. The patient is being treated for a diagnosis of thoracic pain and thoracic facet syndrome. The patient has failed to respond to conservative measures including physiotherapy, medications, and activity modification. The diagnosis has been confirmed with prior injections of local anesthetic. A decision was made to proceed with fluoroscopically-guided thoracic medial branch radiofrequency neurotomy for therapeutic purposes.

The patient was informed of the risks and benefits of the procedure, as well as alternative treatments. The risks include, but are not limited to death, paralysis, allergic reaction, syncope, arrhythmia, cardiac or respiratory arrest, spinal cord injury, worse pain, scar formation, bleeding, epidural hematoma and infection. All questions were answered prior to proceeding. The patient expressed understanding and gave informed written consent.

Preoperative Diagnosis

Thoracic facet pain, thoracic facet syndrome

Postoperative Diagnosis

Same

Procedure Performed

- Radiofrequency ablation of the thoracic medial branches of the right T5, T6 and T7 nerves to denervate the right T6-T7 and T7-T8 thoracic facet joints
- Fluoroscopic guidance/localization.

The patient was taken into the fluoroscopy suite and was placed prone on the procedure table. The patient was prepped and draped in a sterile fashion. All vital signs were monitored prior to, during, and after the procedure. Oxygen saturation was also monitored and noted to be greater than or equal to 94% throughout the procedure. Cardiac monitoring revealed normal sinus rhythm. A grounding pad was then placed on the patient.

The C-arm was positioned so that the T6, T7 and T8 vertebrae were identified. The superficial soft tissues overlying these structures were anesthetized with 1% lidocaine without epinephrine and buffered with sodium bicarbonate as a local anesthetic. At the T6 vertebrae, a 20-gauge 10 cm radiofrequency cannula with a curved, sharp 10-mm active-tip was advanced down via an oblique approach to the site of the traversing medial branch on the transverse process of the vertebra on the right side. This corresponds to the right T5 medial branch nerve. Cannula positioning was done under intermittent fluoroscopic guidance.

At the T7 vertebrae, a 20-gauge 10-cm radiofrequency cannula with a curved, sharp 10-mm active-tip was advanced down via an oblique approach to the site of the traversing medial branch on the transverse process of the vertebra on the right side. This corresponds to the right T6 medial branch nerve. Cannula positioning was done under intermittent fluoroscopic guidance.

At the T8 vertebrae, a 20-gauge 10 cm radiofrequency cannula with a curved, sharp 10-mm active-tip was advanced down via an oblique approach to the site of the traversing medial branch on the transverse process of the vertebra on the right side. This corresponds to the right T7 medial branch nerve. Cannula positioning was done under intermittent fluoroscopic guidance.

Lateral and AP views were obtained to confirm safe and accurate placement. Then, at each level, the radiofrequency needle stylet was replaced by the radiofrequency heating electrode. Impedances were recorded and were noted to be greater than 300 Ω at each level, with adjustments and repeat imaging performed if necessary. Sensory and motor test stimulation at 50 Hz and 2 Hz respectively was performed at each level to ensure no radicular sensations and to obtain maximal multifidi contractions. After stimulation-confirmed correct needle placement and after aspiration was attempted and was negative for return of blood or other fluid, 1 cc of 1% lidocaine without epinephrine was injected at each level. Repeat imaging again demonstrated correct needle placement. Subsequently at each level, standard (nonpulsed) radiofrequency lesioning was done for approximately 90 seconds at 80°C at each level. The lesioning was repeated two times at each level for approximately 90 seconds. At the cessation of the procedure, a small mixture of betamethasone and 1% lidocaine without epinephrine was injected and the needles removed. Radiographs were obtained for documentation purposes.

The patient tolerated the procedure well and was discharged after an appropriate period of observation. If there are any complications, the patient was instructed to call us. The patient is to follow-up with the physician as noted above within 2–3 weeks.

REFERENCES

1. Rengachary SS, Balabhadra RS. Black disc disease: a commentary. Neurosurg Focus. 2002;13(2):E14.
2. Bogduk N. Spinal Diagnostic and Treatment Procedures: Practice Guidelines, 1st edition. San Francisco, CA: International Spine Intervention Society; 2004.
3. Wilson PR. Thoracic facet syndrome—a clinical entity? Pain Supp. 1987;4:S87.
4. Jeffries B. Facet steroid injections. Spine: State of the art review. 1988;2:409-17.
5. Huston CW, Slipman CW, Furman MB, Hasan S, Derby R. Spinal injections. In: Slipman CW, Derby R, Simeone FA, Mayer TG (Eds): Interventional spine: an algorithmic approach. Philadelphia, PA: Saunders Elsevier; 2008. pp. 245-73.
6. Falco FJE, Furman MB. Thoracic zygapophysial joint intra-articular injection, posterior approach. In: Furman MB, Lee TS, Berkwits L (Eds): Atlas of Image-Guided Spinal Procedures. Philadelphia, PA: Elsevier Saunders; 2013. pp. 213-7.
7. Dreyfuss P, Tibiletti C, Dreyer SJ. Thoracic zygapophysial joint pain patterns. A study in normal volunteers. Spine. 1994;19(7):807-11.
8. Fukui S, Ohseto K, Shiotani M. Patterns of pain induced by distending the thoracic zygapophyseal joints. Regional Anesth. 1997;22(4):332-6.

9. Schwarzer AC, Wang SC, O'Driscoll D, et al. The ability of computed tomography to identify a painful zygapophysial joint in patients with chronic low back pain. Spine. 1995;20(8):907-12.
10. van Kleef M, Vanelderen P, Cohen SP, et al. 12. Pain originating from the lumbar facet joints. Pain Pract. 2010;10(5):459-69.
11. Weksler N, Klein M, Gurevitch B, et al. Phenol neurolysis for severe chronic nonmalignant pain: is the old also obsolete? Pain Med. 2007;8(4):332-7.
12. Bogduk N, Wilson AS, Tynan W. The human lumbar dorsal rami. J Anat. 1982;134(Pt 2):383-97.
13. Bogduk N. The innervation of the lumbar spine. Spine. 1983;8(3):286-93.
14. Chua WH, Bogduk N. The surgical anatomy of thoracic facet denervation. Acta Neurochir (Wien). 1995;136(3-4):140-4.
15. Chua WH. Clinical anatomy of the thoracic dorsal rami. BMedSci Thesis. University of Newcastle, Newcastle, Australia; 1994.
16. Atluri S, Datta S, Falco FJ, et al. Systematic review of diagnostic utility and therapeutic effectiveness of thoracic facet joint interventions. Pain Physician. 2008;11(5):611-29.
17. Boswell MV, Colson JD, Sehgal N, et al. A systematic review of therapeutic facet joint interventions in chronic spinal pain. Pain Physician. 2007;10(1):229-53.
18. Bogduk N, Aprill C, Derby R. Diagnostic blocks of synovial joints. In: White AH (Ed): Spine Care, Volume One: Diagnosis and conservative treatment. Mosby, St. Louis; 1995. pp. 298-321.
19. Gray D, Bajwa Z, Warfield C. Facet block and neurolysis. In: Waldman SLR, Ross A, et al (Eds). Interventional pain management. Philadelphia: WB Saunders; 2001. pp. 446-83.
20. Czervionke LF, Fenton DS. Facet joint injection and medial branch block. In: Czervionke LF, Fenton DS (Eds): Image-guided spine intervention. Philadelphia, PA: Saunders Elsevier; 2003. pp. 9-50.
21. Dreyfuss P, Tibiletti C, Dreyer S, et al. Thoracic zygapophysial joint pain: a review and description of an intra-articular block technique. Pain Digest. 1994;4:46-54.
22. Barnsley L, Lord S, Bogduk N. Comparative local anesthetic blocks in the diagnosis of cervical zygapophysial joint pain. Pain. 1993;55(1):99-106.
23. Lord SM, Barnsley L, Bogduk N. The utility of comparative local anesthetic blocks versus placebo-controlled blocks for the diagnosis of cervical zygapophysial joint pain. Clin J Pain. 1995;11(3):208-13.
24. Mehnert MJ, Freedman MK. Update on the role of z-joint injection and radiofrequency neurotomy for cervicogenic headache. PM&R. 2013;5(3):221-7.
25. Manchikanti L, Singh V, Pampati V, et al. Evaluation of the prevalence of facet joint pain in chronic thoracic pain. Pain Physician. 2002;5(4):354-9.
26. Czervionke LF, Fenton DS. Facet denervation. In: Czervionke LF, Fenton DS (Eds): Image-guided spine intervention. Philadelphia, PA: Saunders Elsevier; 2003. p. 51-71.
27. Lord SM, Barnsley L, Bogduk N. Percutaneous radiofrequency neurotomy in the treatment of cervical zygapophysial joint pain: a caution. Neurosurgery. 1995;36(4):732-9.
28. Stolker RJ, Vervest AC, Groen GJ. Percutaneous facet denervation in chronic thoracic spinal pain. Acta Neurochir (Wein). 1993;122(1-2):82-90.

29. Speldewinde GC. Outcomes of percutaneous zygapophysial and sacroiliac joint neurotomy in a community setting. Pain Med. 2011;12(2):209-18.
30. Dreyfuss P, Halbrook B, Pauza K, et al. Efficacy and validity of radiofrequency neurotomy for chronic lumbar zygapophysial joint pain. Spine. 2000;25(10): 1270-7.
31. Smuck M, Crisostomo RA Trivedi K, et al. Success of initial and repeated medial branch neurotomy for zygapophysial joint pain: a systematic review. PM&R. 2012;4(9):686-92.
32. Falco FJE, Steinmetz BD, Furman MB. Thoracic zygapophysial joint nerve (medial branch) radiofrequency neurotomy, posterior approach. In: Furman MB, Lee TS, Berkwits L (Eds): Atlas of Image-Guided Spinal Procedures. Philadelphia, PA: Elsevier Saunders; 2013. pp. 225-9.
33. Haspeslagh S, Van Kleef M. Technique of radiofrequency denervation. In: Slipman CW, Derby R, Simeone FA, Mayer TG (Eds): Interventional spine: an algorithmic approach. Philadelphia, PA: Saunders Elsevier; 2008. p. 275-89.

18

Thoracic Disc Herniation

Arjang Abbasi, Shounuck I Patel, Gautam Malhotra

CHIEF COMPLAINT

A 67-year-old right-handed male presents with 2 months of sudden onset, gradually worsening 8/10 mid-back pain radiating into the left ribs (Fig. 18.1).

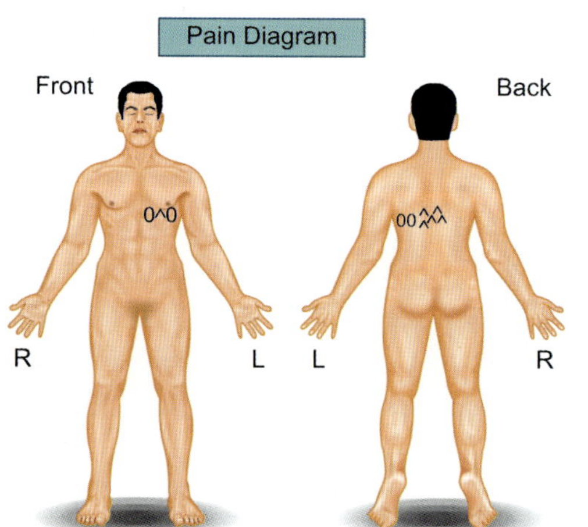

Using the symbols below, the location and type of pain sensations are marked on the diagrams. All the affected areas are included.

TYPE OF SENSATIONS

Aching	^ ^ ^ ^ ^ ^
Burning	X X X X X X
Sharp or stabbing	//////////
Pins and needles	0 0 0 0 0 0
Numbness	II II II II II II

Fig. 18.1: Thoracic disc herniation (Pain diagram)

HISTORY OF PRESENT ILLNESS

He woke up with the symptoms and denies any inciting or traumatic events. He reports that his primary physician ruled out gastrointestinal, renal, cardiac and pulmonary causes. He has already tried nonsteroidal anti-inflammatory medications, acetaminophen, and acupuncture. Chiropractic manipulation of the ribs and thoracic spine did not provide relief. A neurologist ordered diagnostic studies summarized below:

- *X-ray thoracic spine*: mild dextroscoliosis. No osteopenia
- *Magnetic resonance imaging cervical spine with contrast*: mild multilevel degenerative disc disease (DDD)
- *Magnetic resonance imaging thoracic spine with contrast*: multilevel DDD and herniated nucleus pulposus (HNPs) including a large one at T10-11. No intrinsic cord changes (Figs 18.2 and 18.3).

"Shingles" was ruled out. A trial of modalities, manipulation, and lumbar stabilization in physical therapy provided no significant relief. Gabapentin provided some relief but the pain persists. There are no other relieving factors. He denies any identifiable exacerbating factors and specifically denies and worsening with deep inspiration. He denies any associated numbness, tingling, awakening from the pain, weakness, gait difficulties, bladder/bowel dysfunction, unexplained weight loss, fever, chills, night sweats and significant spine surgical/procedural history. The pain is affecting his daily function and quality of life.

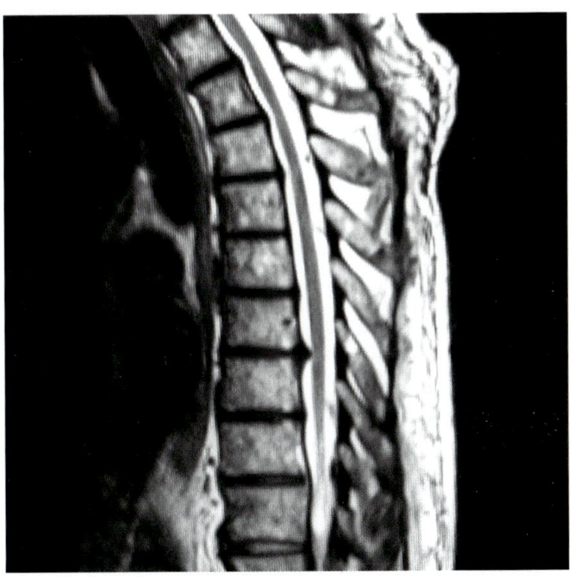

Fig. 18.2: Sagittal image from thoracic spine MRI study with disc herniation visualized at T10-T11

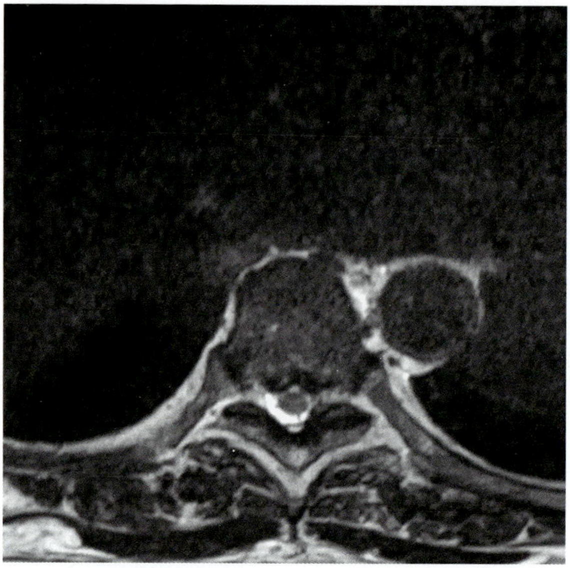

Fig. 18.3: Thoracic spine MRI axial image demonstrating the T10-T11 disc herniation

PAST MEDICAL HISTORY

- Sinusitis
- Colon carcinoma status post-resection
- Diabetes type 2 adult
- Osteoarthritis
- Lysis of adhesions 2005
- Reflux
- Coronary artery disease
- Inguinal hernia status postherniorrhaphy
- Hypertension
- Melanoma

ALLERGIES

No known allergies

FAMILY HISTORY

- Mother and father died in their late 80s due to heart disease.
- Brother has DDD, herniated disc and osteoarthritis.
- Paternal grandmother colon cancer

SOCIAL HISTORY

- *Occupation*: Retired bus operator and classified as disabled through social security/social security disability insurance
- *Living condition*: He is married and has two grown children that have left the home. He lives with his spouse in a single level ranch house with no steps to enter
- *Tobacco*: Former pipe smoker. Quit 2 years ago
- *Alcohol*: Drinks a glass of wine daily

MEDICATION HISTORY

- *Omeprazole*: 20 mg
- *Mobic*: 15 mg
- *Gabapentin*: 600 mg
- *Januvia*: 100 mg
- *Livalo*: 2 mg
- *Diovan HCT*: 160–12.5 mg
- *Allegra allergy*: 180 mg
- *Aspirin*: 81 mg
- Metformin HCL
- Welchol
- *Plavix*: 75 mg
- *Singulair*: 10 mg

REVIEW OF SYSTEMS

- *Constitutional*: See history of present illness
- *HEENT*: denies recent double vision or changes in speech
- *Respiratory*: No shortness of breath or cough
- *Cardiovascular*: See past medical history
- *Gastrointestinal*: See past medical history
- *Genitourinary*: No dysuria, hematuria, incontinence
- *Reproductive*: Negative for dysfunction
- *Metabolic/endocrine:* See past medical history
- *Neurological*: See history of present illness
- *Dermatologic*: No rash or itching
- *Musculoskeletal*: See history of present illness
- *Hematologic*: No easy bruising, bleeding or blood clots
- *Immunologic/allergy*: No environmental allergies
- *Corrective lenses*: Wears glasses.

PHYSICAL EXAMINATION

Vital Signs

- *BP*: 140/90 mm Hg
- *Pulse*: 74/minute
- *Height*: 72 inches
- *Weight*: 180 pounds
- *BMI*: 24.41
- *Head/face/eyes/ears/nose/throat*: Normocephalic. No exophthalmos or nasal deformity. Hearing grossly intact
- *Respiratory*: Normal to inspection
- *Integumentary*: No impressive skin lesions present
- *Psychiatric*: No unusual anxiety noted today.

Neurological

- Manual muscle testing reveals no gross weakness in lower extremities.
- Muscle stretch reflexes are symmetric 2+ in the biceps, triceps, pronator teres, quadriceps, medial hamstring and triceps surae.
- Babinski testing is symmetric and reveals downgoing toes.
- Sensation is symmetric and intact in all dermatomes of the thorax, abdomen, upper and lower limbs.

Thoracic and Lumbar Spine

Inspection

- There is a lateral/anterior abdominal surgical scar.
- There is no thoracic spinal deformity including scoliosis or excessive kyphosis.
- No atrophy noted in the upper or lower limbs.

Palpation

- Mild left-sided paraspinal tenderness without muscle spasm
- No tenderness of the ribs
- There is no spinous process
- No percussive tenderness is elicited.

Range of Motion

- Lumbar active range of motion does not produce pain.
- Intersegmental spine motion during ROM is preserved.

- Right lateral lumbar flexion is 40°, left lateral lumbar flexion is 40°
- Lumbar flexion is 90°, lumbar extension is 35°.

Tone

Normal without velocity-dependent increase with passive range of motion

Stability

Hip motion is painless and within normal limits. Knee exam is normal and painless bilaterally.

Special

Straight leg raise, femoral stretch, Patrick's test, distraction testing and contralateral straight leg raise are negative bilaterally.

ASSESSMENT WITH DIFFERENTIAL DIAGNOSIS

Mid-Back Pain Radiating into Ribs

Differential includes:

- *Neuromuscular*: imaging evidence of herniated nucleus pulposis without myelopathy. This could be causing a thoracic radiculopathy which would explain the symptoms. Diabetes is also a risk factor for thoracic radiculopathy. Shingles, syrinx, and other cord etiologies are unlikely given history and imaging.
- *Musculoskeletal*: rib and spine fracture ruled out. There is a myofascial component but this seems less contributory and more likely a sequelum of underlying cause.
- *Visceral*: renal, cardiac, pulmonary and gastrointestinal causes ruled out already. Neoplastic or paraneoplastic causes should be considered; however, these seem less likely given the presentation and workup thus far.

Treatment Plan

- *Education*: discussed the relevant anatomy and proposed etiology of his pain
- *Physical therapy*: one to two sessions with goals of preventing maladaptive sequelae of pain and providing a home exercise program. This should include posture training, chin tucks, cervical stabilization, ergonomics, scapular retractor strengthening, pectoral stretching and education of modalities to address myofascial pain for home use (e.g. heat, tens, etc.)

- Transforaminal thoracic epidural steroid injection (ESI) left at T10, T11. The patient was instructed to discontinue medications prior to procedure pending clearance from their provider. The risks, benefits, alternatives and expectations of the proposed procedure were discussed at length with the patient, as well as the procedure itself and expected recovery period. The patient was allowed as much time as necessary to ask all appropriate questions and they were answered to the patient's satisfaction. A medication alert sheet was given to the patient instructing the patient to stop the listed medications 1 week prior to procedure.
- *Medication*: he will try tramadol 50 mg in the interim to see if it helps.
- *Follow-up*: next available appointment for spine injection.

BACKGROUND

Thoracic back pain can originate from intervertebral disc disease, facet joints, ligaments, fascia, muscles, and nerves.[1] Neuropathic thoracic flank and/or chest-wall pain can be radicular due to herniated nucleus pulposus, spinal stenosis, or other mechanical nerve root impingement such as from a fracture or metastatic disease. Focal or radiating thoracic pain can also stem from intercostal nerve mononeuropathy.[2] Post-thoracotomy pain syndrome is a possible cause of chronic thoracic pain postoperatively, but is considered separate from thoracic spinal pain.[1]

The prevalence of thoracic back pain has been reported as 5–15%, compared to 24–44% cervical and 33–56% lumbar. Thoracic disc injuries represent 0.25–0.75% of all disc herniations.[3] Although computed tomography, magnetic resonance imaging and postmortem findings have suggested incidence as high as 15.2[4]–37%,[5] it has been stated that more than 70% of thoracic disc herniations are asymptomatic[6] with an incidence of one per million patients.[5] However, symptomatic cases of thoracic disc herniation have been reported at almost all thoracic levels.[7]

Thoracic disc herniation may manifest as myelopathy, radiculopathy, back pain[5] or flank pain,[7] but the presenting symptoms often overlap with pulmonary, cardiac, gastrointestinal or genitourinary etiologies,[8] therefore, thoracic radiculopathy is often a diagnosis of exclusion.

Although thoracic disc degeneration and endplate irregularities are common findings, pain attributed to thoracic disc herniation is considered extremely rare. Since imaging ultimately can only examine anatomy and not physiology, MRI, CT, myelography and radiographs are expectedly as ineffective of identifying pain from disc herniation in the thoracic spine as it is in the lumbar spine.[9] Electrodiagnostic examination can help confirm thoracic radiculopathy as well as differentiate from intercostal nerve mononeuropathy, and somatosensory evoked potentials can be performed for suspected thoracic myelopathy.[7]

INDICATIONS FOR INJECTION

Thoracic epidural steroid injections for radiculopathy are indicated in the presence of image-confirmed disc herniation with or without electrodiagnostic verification, and in the absence of more life-threatening etiologies. Thoracic epidural steroid injections have also been used for acute post-thoracotomy pain.[1]

TREATMENT ALTERNATIVES

Thoracic radiculopathy can be managed conservatively similar to radiculopathy at other spinal levels. Pharmacologic treatment includes nonsteroidal anti-inflammatory, neuropathic, muscle relaxant, and opioid medications. An oral steroid dose pack may be considered for acute radiculopathy. Physical therapy can include spinal extension, spinal stabilization, and posture training. Orthotics may be used and modalities may give short-term symptomatic relief.[7]

Thoracic epidural steroid injections can have an interlaminar or transforaminal approach. Interventional treatments for other causes of thoracic pain may include facet blocks, radiofrequency ablation, intercostal nerve blocks, and thoracic paravertebral blocks.

Surgical interventions range from laminectomy to thoracoscopic discectomy,[5] but there is no consensus on optimal surgical approach.[10]

CONTRAINDICATIONS

There is a relative scarcity of literature regarding epidural steroid injections for thoracic disc herniations as compared with other levels. Contraindications are the same as for other spinal levels such as bleeding disorders, uncontrolled psychiatric disorders, uncontrolled acute or chronic medical illness, pregnant or lactating women, history of adverse reaction to anesthetic, contrast, or steroids. Additional contraindications include patients with higher propensity for pneumothorax including but not limited to those with bullous lung disease and uncontrolled spasms.

THORACIC TRANSFORAMINAL EPIDURAL STEROID INJECTION

Preparation

- Informed consent is obtained.
- Risks and benefits are reviewed with the patient. Risks are similar to other epidural steroid injections, except for the addition of a pneumothorax

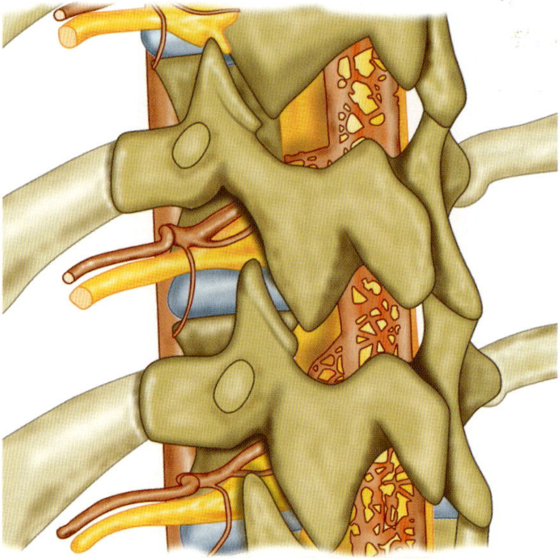

Fig. 18.4: Schematic of a left ipsilateral oblique view of the thoracic spine, demonstrating the target area just below the pedicle of the vertebral body and lateral to the lamina. Note the location of the radicular arteries anterior to the traversing nerve roots

when performing a transforaminal thoracic ESI. Attention should also be paid to the artery of Adamkiewicz given that the pain is left sided and in the thoracic region (Fig. 18.4).

EQUIPMENT AND MEDICATIONS

- Fluoroscope with a C-arm, preferably with digital subtraction angiography. The procedure can be done in an outpatient setting or a hospital setting.
- *The tools include*: 25 gm 3.5 inch spinal needle, sterile procedure tray, low volume connection tube, Appropriate syringes: Two 5 mL syringes; One 3 mL syringe; 18-gauge needle (to draw meds); 25-gauge needle (to inject anesthetic)
- *Medication*: Dexamethasone 10 mg/mL preservative free; Preservative-free 1% lidocaine; nonionic contrast-I use omnipaque.

TECHNIQUE: OBLIQUE SUBPEDICULAR TRANSFORAMINAL APPROACH

- Patient lies prone on a fluoroscopic table with arms above shoulder level. A true AP view of the thoracic spine is obtained to assess the target level counting from the first thoracic level. Once the correct level is identified, the fluoroscope is obliqued ipsilaterally to the point where the lateral margin of the ribs and pedicles are clearly delineated. The target point is

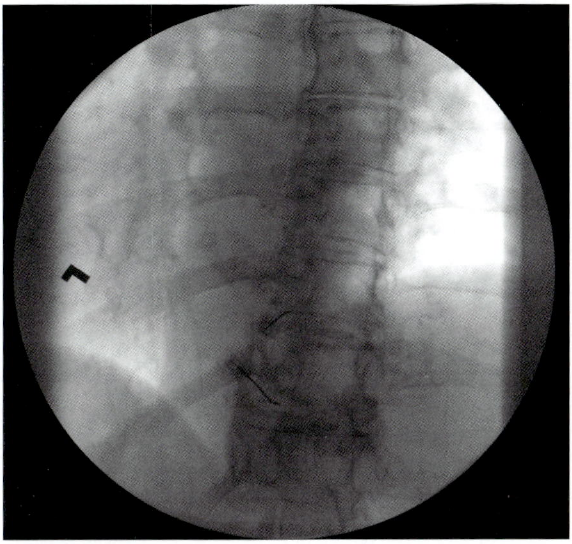

Fig. 18.5: Oblique view with the two needles precontrast. Notice at the left T10 level, the needle was angled a bit more inferiorly due to significant osteoarthritis obstructing the left T10 foramen

the area just below the pedicle and lateral to the lamina. Once the area is identified, the area is anesthetized using 1% lidocaine. A 25-gauge 3.5 inch needle is advanced under live fluoroscopic imaging to the identified area (Fig. 18.5). If the patient identifies any pain that would mimic the pain caused by spinal nerve root irritation, the needle should be withdrawn slightly and reinserted until the optimal position is obtained. The caudal deviation of the needle would increase the chance of contacting the target nerve which traverses caudal to the pedicle. Care should be taken to avoid lateral deviation of the needle to the ribs or medial deviation past the lamina. Needle should be advanced until the needle contact the posterior aspect of the foramen. At that point an AP view is obtained to ensure proper placement of the needle (Fig. 18.6) followed by a lateral view (Fig. 18.7) to ensure adequate placement of the needle. Once the needle is in the optimal position, contrast should be injected under live fluoroscopic guidance to ensure no intravascular or intrathecal flow is obtained (Figs 18.8 and 18.9). If venous uptake is noted, the needle should be repositioned to ensure vascular flow is no longer seen. In case of intra-arterial or intrathecal flow, the procedure should be discontinued. Digital subtraction angiography is recommended if available followed by a test dose of 1% lidocaine in order to ensure lack of any significant vascular uptake. A neurologic exam 90 seconds post-test dose can be done to further ensure lack of any significant vascular uptake.

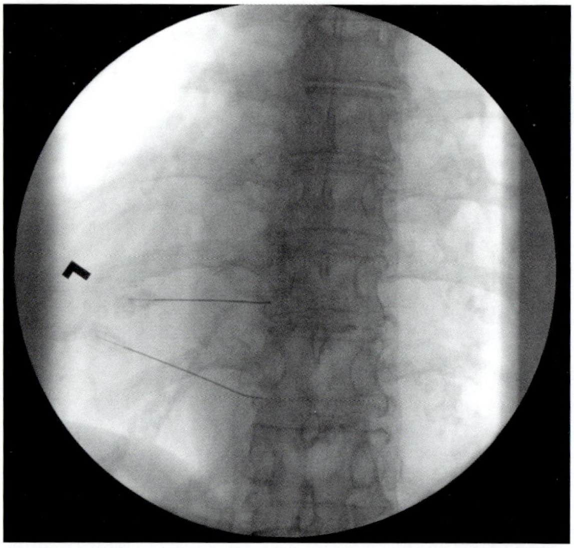

Fig. 18.6: Anteroposterior view. The needle is slowly adjusted if needed in the AP view

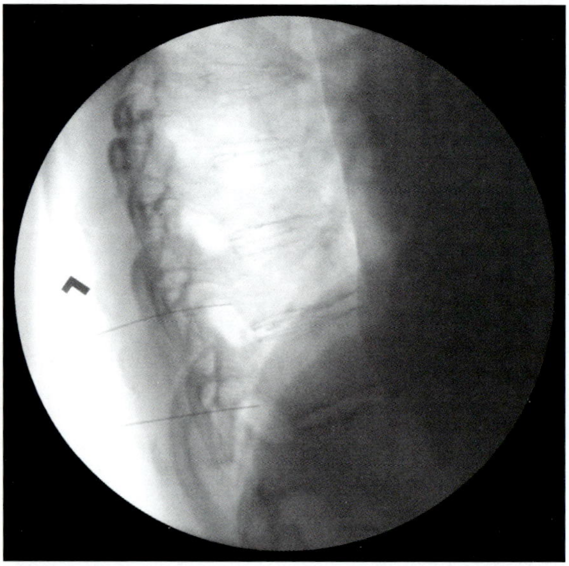

Fig. 18.7: Lateral view. Needle position is confirmed using a lateral view and adjustments are made if necessary

- In this patient's case, the injection was performed at the left T10, T11 levels. A mixture of 15 mg dexamethasone /2.5 mL 1% lidocaine was used, 2.0 mL at each level. This patient tolerated the procedure well with no adverse reactions. Vitals and oxygen saturation were monitored during the procedure.

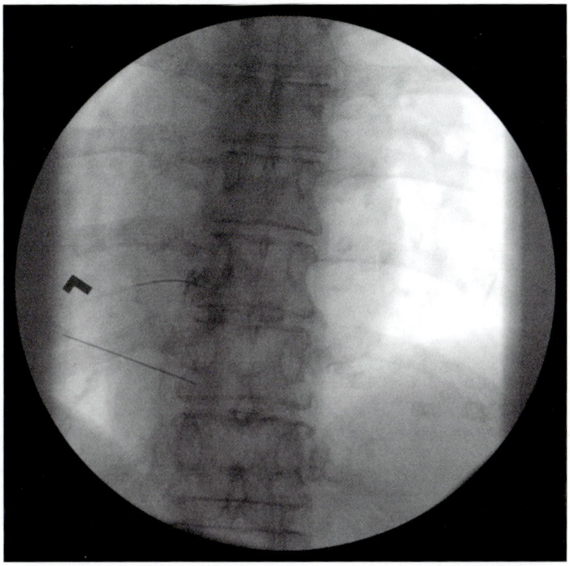

Fig. 18.8: Contrast injected at the left T10 level. Notice the contrast outlining the exiting nerve root and the pedicle

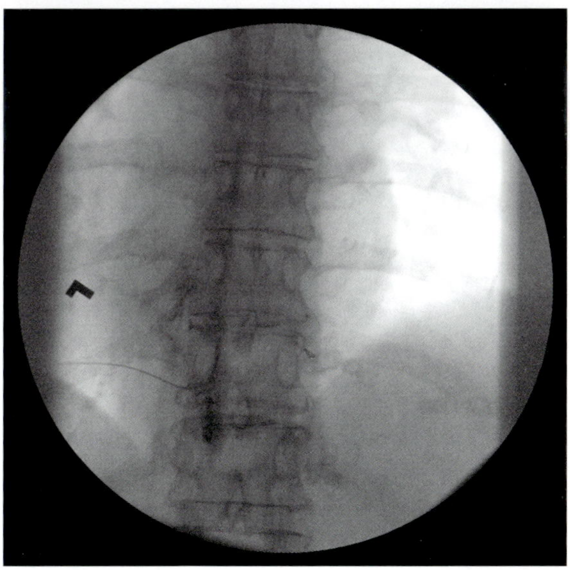

Fig. 18.9: Contrast injected at the left T11 level. Once again, the contrast outlines the exiting nerve root

OTHER TECHNIQUES

- Variable approaches have been described to perform thoracic transforaminal ESIs. This author generally uses the subpedicular oblique approach as described above. Another oblique approach is an infraneural approach where the target point is slightly medial to the head of the rib opposite the foramen—which is below the nerve.[11] A more recent oblique technique has also been described where the needle contacts the posterosuperior aspect of the rib to the lateral aspect of the lamina and then medially, anteriorly toward the neuroforamen.[12] A dorsal approach has also been described where the target point is dorsal to the spinal nerve and the procedure is done entirely in the AP view.[11] With the oblique view, the target is a directly visualized bony landmark. Therefore, the chance of a pneumothorax is theoretically lower compared to the dorsal approach. For this reason, we prefer the oblique view. In addition, direct view of the foraminae using the oblique approach makes the procedure less technically challenging, especially in patients with severe degeneration and facet arthropathy.

- Thoracic interlaminar approach. Alternatively, an interlaminar thoracic epidural steroid injection can also be considered. The procedure would be done in a similar fashion to an interlaminar cervical or lumbar epidural steroid injection where the lamina below the level of entry is first targeted using a paramedian approach using an AP view. Once the lamina is contacted, the needle is redirected into the interlaminar space. At this point, a lateral view is obtained and the needle is slowly advanced using a loss of resistance technique. Contrast is injected to ensure adequate placement and then the medication is injected. Below is an example of a T12-L1 interlaminar epidural steroid injection (Figs 18.10 and 18.11).

In general, we prefer to use the transforaminal approach to more directly deliver the medication to the affected spinal nerve(s) in the intervertebral foramen.

COMPLICATIONS

In the authors' experience, the complications of thoracic transforaminal epidural steroid injections (TFESI) are similar to those described for cervical[13] and lumbar TFESI.[14] One study of thoracic foraminal nerve blocks reports a complication rate of 4.1% with minor adverse events such as light-headedness, local numbness, muscle spasm, vasovagal response and headache, and one major complication of pneumothorax.[15] There are reports of neurological damage following thoracic TFESI, including paraplegia due to particulate steroid embolic injury to the radiculomedullary artery of Adamkiewicz.[16] However, overall incidence of intravascular injection in transforaminal epidural injections is reportedly 8.2% in one study.[17]

Botwin's study of interlaminar thoracic epidural steroid injections reported no major complications and an adverse effects rate of 20.5%. These included increased pain at injection site, facial flushing (5.1%), transient non positional headache, insomnia on the night of the injection, and one episode

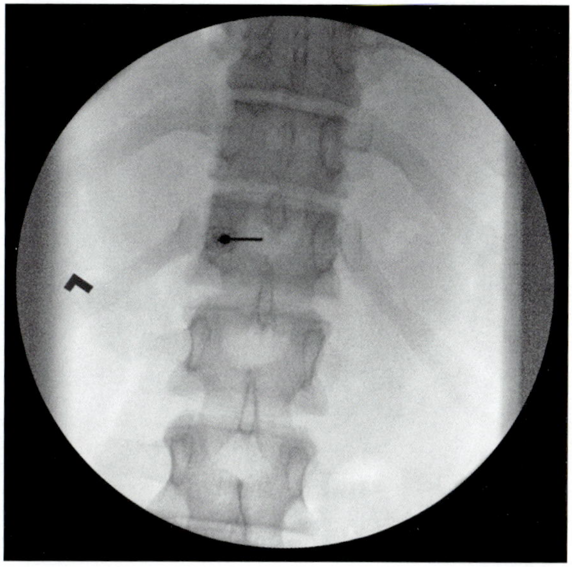

Fig. 18.10: Anteroposterior interlaminar view precontrast. In general, using a paramedian approach, the needle enters the interlaminar space in a 45–60° angle. More the cephalad level, the more angle is needed due to the caudad direction of the spinous process. As we approach the cervical levels, the angle decreases. In this case, the needle was inserted at an almost 90° approach as the patient was moving during the procedure secondary to low pain tolerance. The needle was slowly advanced until the ligamentum flavum was contacted

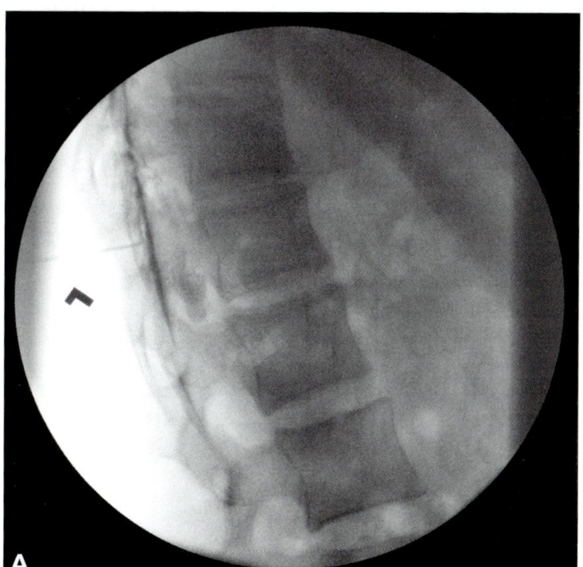

Figs 18.11A

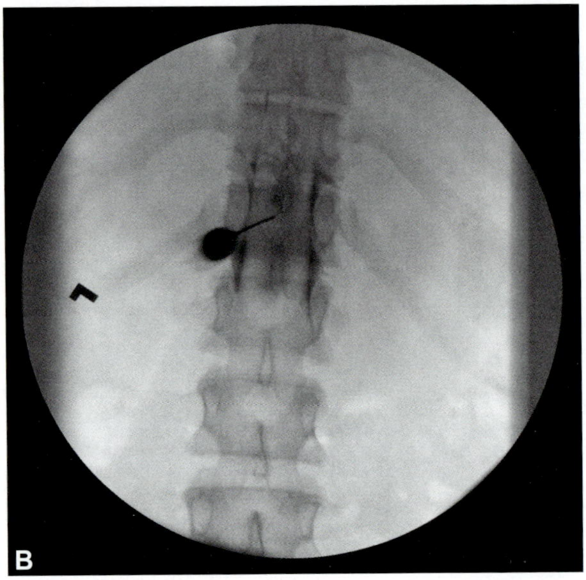

Figs 18.11A and B: Lateral and anteroposterior views—interlaminar T12-L1 ESI post-contrast. (A) Contrast confirms correct placement of the needle in the epidural space in the lateral view; (B) Contrast pattern viewed in the AP view

of fever the night of the procedure.[18] A more recent prospective evaluation of 301 thoracic interlaminar epidural injections revealed intravascular penetration (4%) with return of blood in 2.7% dural punctures (1.3%), vasovagal reactions (0.33%), facial flushing (0.33%), transient spinal cord and nerve root irritation (1% and 0.33%).[19]

EVIDENCE TO SUPPORT THE PROCEDURE

Currently the evidence for thoracic interlaminar and TFESIs in the management of thoracic disc herniations is scant. There is only one prospective study in preliminary support of thoracic interlaminar epidural injections.[1,9] At the time of this publication, no studies could be found regarding thoracic TFESIs. It is, however, considered an appropriate step in management if life-threatening concerns (i.e. neoplasm, infection, rapidly progressive myelopathy, cardiopulmonary etiology, etc.) and appropriate imaging have been addressed, especially with chronic thoracic pain (Benyamin, Wang et al. 2012).[14]

Coding

- 64479: thoracic transforaminal injection
- 64480: additional level/thoracic transforaminal
- 62310: Thoracic interlaminar

REFERENCES

1. Benyamin RM, Wang VC, Vallejo R, et al. A systematic evaluation of thoracic interlaminar epidural injections. Pain Physician. 2012;15(4):E497-514.
2. Santos PS, Resende LA, Fonseca RG, et al. Intercostal nerve mononeuropathy: study of 14 cases. Arq Neuropsiquiatr. 2005;63(3B):776-8.
3. Stout AHN, Kaufman MS. Spinal injection techniques in Physical Medicine & Rehabilitation. Braddom RL (Ed). Saunders: Philadelphia, PA; 2011. pp. 541-62.
4. Uribe JS, Smith WD, Pimenta L, et al. Minimally invasive lateral approach for symptomatic thoracic disc herniation: initial multicenter clinical experience. J Neurosurg Spine. 2012;16(3):264-79.
5. Wait SD, Fox DJ, Kenny KJ, et al. Thoracoscopic resection of symptomatic herniated thoracic discs: clinical results in 121 patients. Spine. 2012;37(1):35-40.
6. Ozturk C, Tezer M, Sirvanci M, et al. Far lateral thoracic disc herniation presenting with flank pain. Spine J. 2006;6(2):201-3.
7. O'Connor RC, Andary MT, Russo RB, et al. Thoracic radiculopathy. Phys Med Rehabil Clin N Am. 2002;13(3):623-44.
8. Papadakos N, Georges H, Sibtain N, et al. Thoracic disc prolapse presenting with abdominal pain: case report and review of the literature. Ann R Coll Surg Engl. 2009;91(5):W4-6.
9. Manchikanti L, Cash KA, McManus CD, et al. A preliminary report of a randomized double-blind, active controlled trial of fluoroscopic thoracic interlaminar epidural injections in managing chronic thoracic pain. Pain Physician. 2010;13(6):E357-69.
10. Deviren V, et al. Minimal invasive anterolateral transthoracic transpleural approach: a novel technique for thoracic disc herniation. A review of the literature, description of a new surgical technique and experience with first 12 consecutive patients. J Spinal Disord Tech. 2011;24(5):E40-8.
11. Bogduk N. Thoracic Transforaminal injections, in Practice Guidelines: Spinal Diagnostic and Treatment Procedures. Bogduk N (Ed). International Spine and Intervention Society: San Francisco, California; 2004. pp. 294-313.
12. Rosas HG, Gilula LA. Performing thoracic transforaminal injections: a new technique. Radiology. 2010;254(2):595-600.
13. Malhotra G, Abbasi A, Rhee M. Complications of transforaminal cervical epidural steroid injections. Spine (Phila Pa 1976). 2009;34(7):731-9.
14. Manchikanti L, Abdi S, Atluri S, et al. An update of comprehensive evidence-based guidelines for interventional techniques in chronic spinal pain. Part II: guidance and recommendations. Pain Physician. 2013;16(2 Suppl):S49-283.
15. Wang A, Pilgram TK, Gilula LA. Immediate complications and pain relief associated with 296 fluoroscopically guided thoracic foraminal nerve blocks. AJR Am J Roentgenol. 2011;197(6): 1410-6.
16. Glaser SE, Shah RV. Root cause analysis of paraplegia following transforaminal epidural steroid injections: the 'unsafe' triangle. Pain Physician. 2010;13(3): 237-44.
17. Nahm FS, Lee CJ, Lee SH, et al. Risk of intravascular injection in transforaminal epidural injections. Anaesthesia. 2010;65(9):917-21.

18. Botwin KP, Baskin M, Rao S. Adverse effects of fluoroscopically guided interlaminar thoracic epidural steroid injections. Am J Phys Med Rehabil. 2006;85(1):14-23.
19. Manchikanti L, Malla Y, Wargo BW, et al. A prospective evaluation of complications of 10,000 fluoroscopically directed epidural injections. Pain Physician. 2012;15(2):131-40.

Index

Page numbers followed by *f* refer to figure.

T

V

W

X